The Physician's Guide To Managed Care

Edited by
David B. Nash, MD, MBA
Director of Health Policy and Clinical Outcomes
Thomas Jefferson University
Philadelphia, Pennsylvania

AN ASPEN PUBLICATION®
Aspen Publishers, Inc.
Gaithersburg, Maryland
1994

Library of Congress Cataloging-in-Publication Data

The Physician's survival guide to managed care/
edited by David B. Nash.
p. cm.

Includes bibliographical references and index.
ISBN 0-08342-0393-6
1. Managed care programs (Medical care)—United States.
2. Medicine—Practice—United States. I. Nash, David B.
[DNLM: 1. Managed Care Programs—United States.
2. Practice Management, Medical. W 275 P475 1994]
RA413.5.U5P48 1994
362.1'0425—dc20
DNLM/DLC
for Library of Congress
93-24024
CIP

Editorial Resources: Ruth Bloom

Library of Congress Catalog Card Number: 93-24024
ISBN: 0-8342-0393-6

Printed in the United States of America

1 2 3 4 5

To the memory of Ernest Saward, MD,
Who taught me what managed care was;

To the Robert Wood Johnson Foundation
Clinical Scholars Program,
That enabled me to see what managed care does;

To the leadership of Thomas Jefferson University,
Who let me dream about what
managed care could mean;

And to Esther Jean Nash
and our children—Leah, Rachel, and Jacob—
Who let me put it all together, always.

Table of Contents

Chapter 7—The Centers of Excellence Phenomena..................**161**
Daniel Dragalin and *Philip D. Goldstein*

Chapter 8—Understanding Your Managed Care Practice:
The Critical Role of Case Mix Systems..........................**189**
Norbert Goldfield

Contributors

Marc A. Bard, MD
Director of Medical Staff Development
Harvard Community Health Plan
Brookline Village, Massachusetts
and
Principle
Marc Bard Management Consultants
West Newton, Massachusetts

Michael W. Cropp, MD
Associate Medical Director
Quality and Utilization Management
Health Care Plan
Buffalo, New York

Daniel Dragalin, MD, MPH
Towers, Perrin
Washington, DC

Kenneth R. Epstein, MD
Clinical Assistant Professor of Medicine
Associate Director
Division of Internal Medicine
Thomas Jefferson University
Philadelphia, Pennsylvania

Daniel H. Friend, MBA
Executive Vice President
National Association of Managed
    Care Physicians
Richmond, Virginia

Norbert Goldfield, MD
Medical Director
3M/H.I.S. Corporation
Wallingford, Connecticut

Philip D. Goldstein, MD, MPH
President/CEO and Medical Director
Holy Redeemer Managed Care
    Organization
Holy Redeemer Health System, Inc.
Huntingdon Valley, Pennsylvania

Susan L. Howell, MSS
Coordinator, Outcomes Projects
Center for Research in
    Medical Education and Health Care
Thomas Jefferson University
Philadelphia, Pennsylvania

Edward F.X. Hughes, MD, MPH
J.L. Kellogg Graduate School of
    Management
and
The Center for Health Services and
    Policy Research
Northwestern University
Evanston, Illinois

Leonard A. Katz, MD
Associate Medical Director
Health Care Plan
and
Professor of Medicine
School of Medicine and Biomedical
    Sciences
State University of New York at Buffalo
Buffalo, New York

John La Puma, MD
General Internist
The Nesset Health Center
Park Ridge, Illinois
and
Consultant in Clinical Ethics
Lutheran General Hospital
Park Ridge, Illinois
and
Clinical Associate Professor of Medicine
University of Chicago Hospitals
    and Clinics
Chicago, Illinois

Harry L. Leider, MD, MBA
Health Center Director, Boston Center
Harvard Community Health Plan
and
Instructor of Medicine
Harvard Medical School
Boston, Massachusetts

Alan H. Rosenstein, MD, MBA
Vice President
Clinical Information
HBOC & Company
Atlanta, Georgia

David Schiedermayer, MD
Associate Professor of Medicine
Division of General Internal Medicine
Medical College of Wisconsin
Milwaukee, Wisconsin

David J. Shulkin, MD
Director
Clinical Outcome Assessment and
   Quality Management
and
Assistant Professor of Medicine
University of Pennsylvania Medical
Center
Philadelphia, Pennsylvania

R. S. Venable,
   MD, FAAFP, FACEP
Chief Medical Officer
Humana Health Plan-Tampa Bay
Tampa, Florida

William C. Williams III, MD
Chief of Staff
Richmond Health Care Group
   (Family Practice)
and
President
National Association of Managed
   Care Physicians
Richmond, Virginia

Foreword

When the history of late twentieth century American health care is written, the growth and development of managed care will undoubtedly be the singular feature of that history. The presence of managed care distinguishes the delivery of health care in the United States from that of any other nation. This presence guarantees that our approach to the pressing dual challenge of expanding access and moderating costs will be unique among all the nations of the world.

Thus, the timing of this book by Dr. Nash and his talented colleagues could not be better. Health care providers, particularly physicians, function in a world increasingly altered and dominated by managed care. The challenges posed by managed care to this generation of providers are unique and without precedent. Accordingly, the solutions to these challenges will, per force, be unique and evolve experientially through a process of learning. It is to assist physicians to identify and surmount these challenges in a professionally and socially responsible manner that this book is written.

Central to a successful response to the challenges of managed care is an understanding of what it is. Interestingly, managed care is one of the most commonly used terms in any discussion of current health care, but it is rarely defined. When attempts are made to define it, they range from statements that "it can't be defined," to listings of the "things" that make up managed care. These listings generally order the "things" of managed care along a spectrum, from the least intrusive forms of managed care—for example, indemnity insurance with a pre-admission certification rider—to the most centralized, the staff model HMO. What is needed, however, is a conceptual definition of managed care. In order to set a context for the various challenges posed by managed care, which are covered in this book, I would like to offer such a definition:

> *Managed care is the process of the application of standard business practices to the delivery of health care in the traditions of the American free enterprise system.*

First and foremost, managed care is a "process." It is change itself. The "things" of managed care, with the exception of the first generation of staff and group model HMOs, are the results of this process, not the cause. The application of standard business practices to the delivery of health care refers to the the effect of Adam Smith's invisible hand on an industry that heretofore has been decentralized, unorganized, and—for those who hold a pejorative view—*dis*organized. The process involves the economic disciplining of this industry, as all other American industries have to date been disciplined. This exercise forces surplus, excess, and waste out of the industry and into other more productive social endeavors. Managed care is doing this to health care.

The final component of the definition stresses that this process is in the traditions of the American free enterprise system. I emphasize this point because many American physicians, in their hearts, still believe that an HMO is the last remaining agent of the international communist conspiracy. Yet the process is pure capitalism. And, as the citizens of Eastern Europe are now discovering, capitalism is not a warm, fuzzy thing. It is a strict disciplinarian, and there are winners and losers.

There have been two driving forces in the process of managed care. The first derives from those who see this process as a chance "to do it better." I call this the professional force. The second force comprises those who see this process as a chance to make money. I call this the pecuniary force. The two are inextricably linked and are often at war with each other in managed care organizations. A managed care organization cannot survive without the pecuniary force because there will be no bottom line. Similarly, it cannot survive without the professional force because The organization will ultimately lose its social purpose and be forced out of business. In assessing managed care organizations, it is important to determine which force is in the ascendancy—the dominant force—in the organization. *The Physician's Guide to Managed Care* provides many fine norms and examples of how to maximize this professional force in managed care organizations, appropriately channel the pecuniary force, and avoid inappropriate dominance by it.

The *sine qua non* of the process of managed care is the diffusion of management across a sector of our economy where management has not previously been a paramount presence—management that makes decisions regarding the appropriate mix of the factors necessary to produce a product, in this case, the health care of a defined population; that negotiates prices for factors of production in ways not previously possible; that strives, as do all managers in all other industries, to achieve the best quality product for the least cost; and that systematically measures and seeks to continuously improve the outcomes of that product. This book provides a manual for physicians on how to achieve these goals in the new and critically important sector of managed care, the sector that will dominate the future of the delivery of health care in this nation.

Edward F. X. Hughes, MD, MPH
J. L. Kellogg Graduate School of Management and
The Center for Health Services and Policy Research
Northwestern University
Evanston, Illinois

Acknowledgments

Any multiauthored, edited text requires an unusual amount of teamwork to weave together the seemingly unrelated efforts of many talented individuals. I am therefore grateful to all of my colleagues who contributed chapters to this unique book, and to Ms. Susan Howell, my research associate. Susan worked with each author, gently but unrelentingly, shepherding them through multiple drafts of each chapter. She was unflappable in her temperament and thoroughly professional in all her dealings with the contributors. There would not have been a book without her.

Of course, I was able to undertake the editorship of this project only because of the strong and enthusiastic leadership provided by my two University bosses—Thomas J. Lewis, senior vice president of Health Administration and chief executive officer of Thomas Jefferson University Hospital, and Joseph S. Gonnella, MD, senior vice president of Academic Affairs and dean of Jefferson Medical College. Their expressed confidence in me is a source of continued energy.

Jack Bruggeman, my editor at Aspen, had a hunch nearly three years ago that a broad market existed for such a book. I hope that time will prove him right. Jack was a patient and unobtrusive editor, exercising his insights at critical junctures in the project.

Elizabeth Brown, my executive administrative assistant, organized everything and ensured our collective timeliness. She is a veteran of other scholarly skirmishes, having been at my side for three books and dozens of journal manuscripts.

Way back in 1978, Mitch Greenlick, PhD and Don Freeborn, PhD of the Kaiser Foundation Health Services Research Center in Portland, Oregon; and Robert Berg, MD and Bill Barker, MD of the

University of Rochester School of Medicine and Dentistry granted me the opportunity to see firsthand one of the greatest managed care organizations in the country—before most clinicians even knew what the term health maintenance organization (*HMO*) meant. In retrospect, I guess they started it all for me!

Finally, my enduring love and gratitude go to my physician wife, Esther Jean Rolnick Nash and our children—twin daughters Leah Brooke and Rachel Susan, and son Jacob Philip, for their support and understanding. As I continue to balance the many priorities in my busy life, they remain unassailably first and foremost.

David B. Nash, MD, MBA
Philadelphia, PA

Chapter 1

Overview

David B. Nash

Once vilified by mainstream American medicine as an inevitable road to socialism, managed care by all accounts is now the mainstream. At least half of all practicing physicians have become involved in one or more managed care arrangements, and physicians have accepted the trade-off of lower fees for a guaranteed flow of patients.[1] How we arrived at this state of affairs is fascinating history, and the reader is referred to the burgeoning literature about managed care, especially our sister Aspen publication, *The Managed Care Handbook* (second edition) by Peter Kongstvedt.

The goal of this book, however, is not to retrace Dr. Kongstvedt's steps but rather to provide clinicians at all levels of training and experience with a glimpse into the future. What will it be like to work in a managed care environment through the next decade—especially under any number of national health care reform proposals? Will the continued erosion of professional autonomy[2] render physicians more susceptible to the "White Coat-Blue Collar Syndrome?"[3]

Physicians have come a long way from printing bumper stickers reading, "Say No to HMO." Moreover, "before doctors reject managed care as too interventionist, they should consider the probable alternatives. In the future, they are likely to face a choice between centralized government regulatory mechanisms, including global budgets, and individual incentives for cost control that operate in a pluralistic, privately dominated system. *The status quo is not a viable option."*[1]

If we accept the notion that the status quo is in fact not viable, we must then be adequately prepared to meet these future challenges. This book fills in some of the gaps in medical education that has left clinicians ill-prepared to contend with capitated payment systems, teamwork, a strong emphasis on practice guidelines and patient outcomes, profiles of their practices, and closer scrutiny by employers and third-party payers.[4]

Yet, I am not presumptuous enough to contend that this single volume is sufficient preparation. Doctors are obligated to keep abreast of changes in the financing and delivery of health services in much the same way that they struggle to remain current with medical advances. In addition to Kongstvedt's aforementioned work, clinicians should regularly review managed care and group practice journals such as *HMO Practice*, published by the HMO Group (in New Brunswick, New Jersey), *Managed Care Quarterly*, edited by Peter Boland and published by Aspen in Gaithersburg, Maryland, and *Medical Group Management Association*, published in Denver, Colorado. Both scholarly peer-reviewed articles and news items will contribute to one's overall education about managed care.

Now, turning to those gaps in medical education, how do we start to fill them in? I will first briefly review some of the basic definitions and vocabulary of managed care to provide a context from which a series of challenges can be viewed. I then examine issues such as the quality of medical services in the managed care setting, the organizational context of physicians' work, the future of medical education in managed care settings, and conclude with a discussion of national health reform and new technologies. Relevant chapters in the text are referred to at the end of each brief section.

MANAGED CARE SYSTEMS

Characteristics and Typology

There are many types of managed care plans, but in general, all of them attempt to integrate the delivery and financing of care and apply new constraints on encounters between physicians and patients.[1] The key constraint for doctors is the limitation placed on the autonomy of their clinical decisions. The constraint for patients is the requirement that they see only physicians who are members of a plan's panel—either a closed or partially open selection of providers.

The financial incentives for patients and providers are somewhat murkier. Patients pay a penalty, or surcharge, to go out of the system to non-plan providers. Physicians, on the other hand, have now assumed some financial risks, fundamentally altering their role "from advocacy to allocation."[5]

Researchers have begun to form a typology for managed care systems as financing and delivery schemes become increasingly complex.[6] Five distinguishing characteristics have been identified:

1. The basic method by which physicians are paid for primary care services (salary, capitation, or fee-for-service).
2. Whether HMO physicians see only HMO patients or whether they also see fee-for-service patients covered by traditional indemnity insurance.
3. The nature of the HMO's financial contract with any existent middle tier.
4. The nature of the risk or reward to primary care physicians, in addition to the basic payment method.
5. The size and nature of the risk pool used to share the risk or reward.

Arguably, these characteristics are not exhaustive and such a discussion is beyond the scope of this book. However, it is incumbent upon clinicians to maintain a certain level of understanding and facility with the core concepts of open and closed panels, incentives, and the like. This topic is discussed further in the chapters that follow.

Finally, managed competition, which some believe is distinct from managed care, refers to a system of health insurance wherein sponsors attempt to affect competition by tying defined contributions to the cost of a least expensive plan that provides coverage for a basic set of benefits. In general, managed competition proposals have sought to expand access as well as institute mechanisms for cost control. Employer mandates are common, though not universal, among managed competition plans.[7] This topic is covered in detail by Dr. Ken Epstein in Chapter 9.

Quality of Care

There remain some skeptics who argue, quite unconvincingly in my view, that the quality of care in managed care settings is not equivalent to care in the private practice, fee-for-service sector. Allow me to lay this argument to rest.

There are no peer-reviewed studies in reputable journals that support this contention. Anecdotes abound, but documentation is not forthcoming. In fact, extensive health services research, conducted by major investigative teams, paints quite a different picture!

Overwhelmingly, the published evidence supports the notion that the quality of care in the managed care arena equals, if not surpasses, the care in the private practice, fee-for-service sector. Quality has been measured across different populations with outcome variables ranging from adherence to federally derived guidelines for immunizations, to blood pressure control, and inpatient care for cancer.[8,9,10] In the last year alone, new studies confirmed the superiority of managed care-based services for older patients with acute myocardial infarction,[11] and men with advanced prostatic cancer.[12] In short, delivering medical services in a managed care setting might enable clinicians to do a *better* job, supported by a network of ancillary personnel, sophisticated tracking systems for pharmaceuticals, and a strong commitment to ongoing quality improvement activities. The collegiality and professional support of a group practice, managed care model might enable peer review to take a more active, nonpunitive position vis-à-vis fee-for-service care.[13]

Purchasers of medical care are convinced that the managed care model will enable them to secure a greater value for their health care dollars. Here, value means the best possible cost-effective care at a competitive price. The business literature abounds with articles describing new alliances between managed care organizations and purchasers working together to pressure hospitals to encourage more efficient care and more parsimonious use of limited resources.[14]

Managed care clinicians might find themselves at the forefront of activities designed to force hospitals to divulge unprecedented amounts and types of information about hospital performance. As managed care networks grow, their market clout will correspondingly increase, enabling them to put "outcomes management" into action in the marketplace. (For a more detailed discussion of this phenomenon, see Nash and Markson.[15])

Readers interested in acquiring the necessary skills to deliver care with value should consult Chapter 6 by Drs. Shulkin and Rosenstein, as well as Chapter 8 on case mix measurement and management by Dr. Goldfield. Chapter 7, by Drs. Dragalin and Goldstein, describes the quality-driven programs already in place nationwide.

Organizational Context of Physicians' Work

The current socialization process of medical school creates physicians ill-prepared to function in an organizational context characterized by hierarchical controls, teamwork responsibilities, and a requirement to surrender some professional autonomy for "the greater good" of the organization. Older physicians (50 or more years of age) may find it difficult or nearly impossible to adapt to a managed care organization—especially a tightly run group or staff model health maintenance organization (HMO). These physicians matured during medicine's "Golden Era," a time without the constraints of prospective payment (diagnosis-related groups [DRGs]), utilization review, and preadmission certification. This group will no doubt bristle at attempts by managed care to impose various clinical algorithms, rules,[16] or worksite productivity standards.

Indeed, astute observers note that many physicians paint all managed care organizations with the same brush: they are indistinguishable due to an across-the-board decrease in professional autonomy![17] Other physicians have maligned the advertising practices of some managed care organizations, labeling them as unethical and, at best, misleading.[18]

Hillman and colleagues have studied the relationship between various financial incentives and physician behavior in the managed care setting.[16] Not surprisingly, they found that doctors respond to financial incentives, or penalties, in the expected direction. The relationship between incentives and quality of care is complex but essentially, if physicians are penalized financially for conducting too many diagnostic tests, they will order fewer tests! Ultimately, patient outcomes have been found to be no different than in the private practice, fee-for-service sector.

Also, some managed care organizations report high physician turnover rates, upwards of 12 percent annually, especially among younger physicians just out of residency and fellowship training programs.[4] How can we explain this observation? Again, even younger doctors, those who never witnessed the "Golden Era," are unaccustomed to working as salaried employees (in group and staff model HMOs). Perhaps the managed care culture's expectations of close working relationships with ancillary professionals, lack of hire and fire authority of individual clinicians (for support personnel), and taboos regarding traditional animosity toward administrators creates an intolerable source of frustration for some. Is all lost then?

I submit that many physicians will increasingly turn to managed care to free them from the administrative hassles of fee-for-service private practice. Others will enjoy abandoning their voluntary staff committee membership with its cumbersome decision-making structure, slavish adherence to consensus, and internecine politics. Managed care will initiate real credentialing[17] for cost-effectiveness based on a true performance assessment[19] rather than contracting with any practitioner willing to discount his or her fees.

Managed care organizations have a responsibility to create better opportunities for continuing medical education. Undoubtedly, they will be the first to take advantage of rapidly developing instructional technologies such as CD-ROMs, interactive videodiscs, teleconferencing, and the like.

Furthermore, managed care organizations may begin to demonstrate the interest, managerial competence, and political will[17] necessary to implement large scale, innovative, educational intervention programs. Such programs would, for example, examine the use of physician "prompts" to order the appropriate antibiotic, or to follow mutually agreed algorithms for the approach to an abnormal pap smear. In short, I believe that primary care physicians in managed care will have unique opportunities and resources enabling them to simultaneously improve quality and lower costs. The price of progress is the surrender of a marginal degree of professional autonomy.

Interested readers should refer to Chapter 3 by Drs. La Puma and Schiedermayer, which examines the ethical dilemmas raised by the issues of incentives, rules, and autonomy. Drs. Leider and Bard present the managerial perspective in Chapter 4 while Chapter 2 by Drs. Katz and Cropp presents the rank and file view of work within the characteristic organizational settings. Hopefully, these chapters will become the framework for a required basic-science like curriculum in managed care for all current medical school sophomores.

Medical Education and National Health Reform

Nearly 15 years ago, academic medical centers and managed care organizations (then exclusively referred to as HMOs) flirted with each other, suspicious of each other's motives and long-term goals. HMO medical directors petitioned academic chiefs of medicine to send trainees to practice at their outpatient sites. The chiefs generally were reluctant. Among their concerns were a lack of appropriate credentials of the HMO staff physicians, the absence of a core ambulatory care curriculum, and a general sense that HMOs may be only another administrative flash in the pan, like "Management by Objectives" and other popular, early 1980s manage-babble.

How things have changed—for all concerned parties! Now, academic departments of medicine, family medicine, pediatrics, and others are looking for enhanced outpatient-based experiences for their trainees. Residency Review Committees (RRC), one arm of the accrediting process for training programs, today mandate increased exposure to all aspects of ambulatory care. The flirtations of the past may result in an arranged marriage of convenience for the near future!

Deep-seated suspicions remain, however. Academicians claim that managed care concepts like "appropriateness," "cost-effectiveness," and "practice protocols" imply research bases, but that their foundations are weak. "Managed care plans' attempts to develop these tools may result from physician leadership or may challenge physicians' judgment about what is best. As more physicians enter into multiple contractual arrangements, in order to sustain a viable practice, autonomy continues to erode. How these developments create inroads into medical education, as a remaining bastion of physician control, therefore becomes a key question."[20]

In addition to the issue of curricular hegemony, the revenue sources for continued support of Graduate Medical Education (GME) add to the aforementioned suspicions. Medicare currently pays hospitals for the costs of GME, which include both direct (salaries) and indirect (they take care of "sicker" patients) components. As a result, payment for all trainees favors inpatient tertiary services over primary care and prevention. Where then will the monies come from to support training in managed care settings, after the stakeholders agree that such training is necessary?

Clearly, a new cooperative spirit must supplant these deeply held suspicions. Some managed care leaders have taken up the challenge. These settings emphasize prevention, primary care, and efficient delivery, as well as exposure of students to generalist role models, and opportunities to conduct community-based research. At the Harvard Community Health Plan in Boston, Massachusetts,[21] the managed care site provides teaching hospitals with access to clinical settings.

At the George Washington University HMO in Washington, DC,[22] even first- and second-year medical students are exposed to the principles of managed care early in their careers. Residents provide reimbursable patient care services, just as in the hospital. Residents are encouraged to participate in areas of research such as decision-analysis and cost-effectiveness of care, and to serve on administrative committees that confront issues like quality assessment, among others.

Other leaders have called for an intellectual overhaul of the current efforts at quality improvement.[23] The managed care environment might be ideally suited to enhance curricular reform in content areas such as

- organization and management
- health systems
- quality theory and methods
- management information systems
- governmental policy
- economics and finance.

If doctors really *can* "negotiate a settlement between themselves and society"[24] to create lasting health care reform, managed care practitioners will be at the forefront of these changes. Please see Chapter 9 by Dr. Epstein, which outlines in detail the proposals for national health care reform.

One must recognize, I believe, that physicians in some managed care organizations are already well along the road to reform and have even staked out some of the moral high ground. For example, in many HMOs, doctors have lived within a "global budget" for decades. They have exchanged an explicit salary scale for less meddling in their day-to-day affairs. Perhaps we can all learn from their experience.

While the editorialists at the *New York Times*[25] claim that managed competition is the answer, they have yet to make the important connection between managed competition and medical education. Simply, I believe we must work to end the dichotomy between managed competition and the need for the training of more primary care practitioners—and the current orientation toward subspecialty fellowships (and hard dollar support for them). The way to launch managed competition is to reorient medical education, in some settings at least, toward primary care. Also, we must pay primary care practitioners higher salaries after training, rather than tinker with the indirect and direct components of GME. Senior medical students will not choose careers in primary care because their *house staff* salaries for three years will be slightly increased, or because positions will be more plentiful.

As previously mentioned, clinicians in managed care settings may be well positioned to take advantage of the burgeoning technology in so-called patient-centered feedback systems.[26] While new opportunities in GME certainly will be available, video-guided patient decision-making tools could make managed care practice more rewarding and fun. Managed care groups could conceivably help practitioners forge a new doctor-patient relationship free of burdens such as cost, access, time, and administrative hassles.

CONCLUSION

The vocabulary of managed care is sometimes needlessly complex and redundant. The opportunities to improve the quality of care, while controlling costs, are real and must be grasped. The organizational context of day-to-day clinical work will continue to be studied, and its relationship to *physician* performance and satisfaction further elucidated. The connections among medical education, current managed care practice, and national health care reform are tenuous now, but will be strengthened in the coming decade. Managed care practitioners will have an enviable number of practice options from which to choose, many enriched by outstanding support systems, continuously working to improve daily performance.

Who should read this book? I believe this multiauthored volume speaks to physicians at all levels of training and experience with a serious interest in practicing within any number of managed care models.

This book is not a primer on HMOs. Because it was written almost exclusively by doctors for doctors, I believe it offers a unique, single-source opportunity to thoroughly evaluate the status of managed care practice, well into the next decade. The end of each chapter contains a pithy commentary by Susan Howell and me that outlines the main points. The commentaries attempt to weave together the different aspects of our tapestry, coalescing the numerous new ideas into a context for further review and analysis.

It is not a political document in that it treats the history and development of managed care in a somewhat cursory manner, preferring instead to examine in detail the organizational context of physicians' work and the implications for professional autonomy. I hope it begins to fill some of the obvious lacunae in medical education and helps to prepare a future generation of physician leaders for the managed care industry.

REFERENCES

1. Iglehart JK. Health policy report: the American health care system: managed care. *N Engl J Med.* 1992;327:742–747.

2. Starr P. *The Social Transformation of American Medicine.* New York:Basic Books;1982.

3. Nash DB, ed. *Future Practice Alternatives in Medicine.* 2nd ed. New York: Igaku-Shoin;1993.

4. Kent C, ed. Doctors and managed care: a rocky road to accommodation. *Medicine and Health-Perspectives.* November 23, 1992.

5. Mechanic D. *From Advocacy to Allocation: The Evolving American Health Care System.* New York: Free Press; 1986.

6. Welch WP, Hillman AL, Pauly MV. Toward new typologies for HMOs. *Milbank Q.* 1990;68:221–243.

7. AMA House of Delegates. Interim Annual Meeting; November 17, 1992; Nashville, Tenn.

8. Ware JE, Brook RH, Rogers WH, et al. Comparison of health outcomes at a health maintenance organization with those of fee-for-service care. *Lancet.* 1986;1:1017–1022.

9. Greenwald HP. HMO membership, co-payment, and initiation of care for cancer: a study of working adults. *Am J Public Health.* 1987;77:461–466.

10. Rossiter LF, Langwell K, Wan TTH, et al. Patient satisfaction among elderly enrollees and dis-enrollees in medicare health maintenance organizations. *JAMA.* 1989; 262:57–63.

11. Carlisle DM, Siu AL, Keeler EB, et al. HMO vs fee-for-service care of older persons with acute myocardial infarction. *Am J Public Health.* 1992;82:1626–1630.

12. Greenwald HP, Henke CJ. HMO membership, treatment, and mortality risk among prostatic cancer patients. *Am J Public Health.* 1992;82:1099–1104.

13. Eisenberg JM, Kabcenell A. Organized practice and the quality of medical care. *Inquiry.* 1988;25:78–89.

14. Jordahl G. HMOs and employers unite to collect outcomes data. *Business and Health.* June 1992:44–50.

15. Nash DB, Markson LE. Outcomes management: the perspective of the players. *Frontiers Health Serv Mngt.* 1991;8:3–51.

16. Hillman AL. Managing the physician: rules versus incentives. *Health Affairs.* 1991; 10:138–146.

17. Berenson RA. A physician's view of managed care. *Health Affairs.* 1991;10:106–119.

18. Brett AS. Sounding board—the case against persuasive advertising by health maintenance organizations. *N Engl J Med.* 1992;326:1353–1356.

19. Nash DB, Markson LE, Howell S, Hildreth EA. Evaluating the competence of physicians in practice: from peer review to performance assessment. *Academic Medicine.* 1993; 68(2):S19–S22.

20. Matherlee KR, Jones JM. Generalist physicians in managed care settings: a different twist on physician education and primary care. George Washington University, Washington, DC, National Health Policy Forum. Issue Brief #597. June 24, 1992.

21. Moore GT. Health maintenance organizations and medical education: breaking the barriers. *Academic Medicine.* 1990;65(7):427–432.

22. Ott JE. Medical education in a health maintenance organization: the George Washington University health plan experience. *HMO/PPO Trends.* 1992;5:6–11.

23. Ziegenfuss JT. Managed care: the strategic future for education in quality. *J Insurance Medicine.* 1992;24:14–19.

24. Welch HG, Fisher ES. Let's make a deal: negotiating a settlement between physicians and society. *N Engl J Med.* 1992;327:1312–1315.

25. Anonymous. The answer: managed competition for America's health. *New York Times.* (Editorial). December 2, 1992.

26. Weinstein MM. Dr. Video—How best to decide what patients need. *New York Times.* (Editorial). December 13, 1992.

Chapter 2

Life of the HMO Physician

Leonard A. Katz
Michael W. Cropp

INTRODUCTION

With the participation of over 18,000 full-time physicians, staff and group model HMOs can no longer be viewed as novel or unusual. Practice in HMOs is a unique—though far from new—departure from traditional solo or small group fee-for-service practice. Historically, the two trends, group practice and prepayment, developed independently, then merged and became what was initially termed *prepaid group practice*. Eventually, prepaid group practice became known as the staff or group model HMO.[1]

In the earliest days, HMO physicians perceived their work as an idealistic participation in a changing world of medical practice. Elimination of the concern about the patient's ability to pay led some physicians to take a chance with a very new movement. Increasingly, the prepaid group practice movement is believed to have the potential to transform the face of medical practice in this country. Medical leaders such as Arnold Relman,[2] former editor of the *New England Journal of Medicine*, and James Todd, executive director of the American Medical Association, have begun to recognize the contributions being made by managed care, and its potential as a model for change.

This chapter strives to define the distinctions between this form of medical practice and traditional fee-for-service, and to convey a sense of what it is like to practice in an HMO. Practice structure, medical staff organization, physician responsibilities, and career opportunities will be addressed. In its full expression, managed care gives the practicing physician the opportunity to participate in a movement that will make medical practice a more rational, conservative, and patient-focused endeavor. John Wennberg of Dartmouth Medical School (Hanover, New Hampshire) recently challenged HMOs to become "islands of rationality" in an environment noted for significant elements of irrationality, and which Wennberg describes as "the sea of supplier-induced demand."[3]

Other significant issues addressed by this chapter include those concerning physician practice within staff and group model HMOs. While the prepaid group practice environment is distinctive, some principles can be applied to the growing number of prepaid insurance programs, such as Independent Practice Associations (IPAs), Preferred Provider Organizations (PPOs), and Exclusive Provider Arrangements (EPAs).

PRACTICE IN AN HMO

The physician practicing in an HMO will undoubtedly encounter a subtle tension between tradition-entrenched "classical" medical practice, and the novelty and challenge offered by the HMO setting. Dissatisfactions and concerns of physicians practicing in HMO settings can emerge because of the "clash of cultures" (described by Harry Leider and Marc Bard in Chapter 4) and the perceived limits of clinical autonomy can be frustrating and difficult to adjust to.

While review of clinical decision making is needed to assure high-quality, effective care, the mechanism of review will vary with the organizational type. Staff and group model HMOs rely heavily on physician peer review for criteria development and retrospective analysis, while IPAs and PPOs tend to rely more on rules, nurse reviewers, and financial incentives. The sense of clinical freedom that emerges in group practice HMOs is a major positive feature for physicians.

Physicians who have previously practiced in a fee-for-service setting recognize the high level of comparability. Angel Gutierrez, MD, an internist who left fee-for-service practice after 17 years states, "I am frequently asked why I left private practice. It doesn't feel as though I left. Actually, even in my fee-for-service practice, I believed that the HMO concept was a sound one, especially in that it could provide me with the freedom to be involved in patient care without having to worry about the logistics of billing and the business side of practice."[4] Family physician Thomas Sheehan, MD, concludes, "I still care for my patients as I did before; that is, the patient and his medical condition and welfare came first. Contrary to many of my colleagues' dire predictions prior to my joining an HMO, I am not told how to practice medicine; I am still a strong advocate for the patient and medical decisions concerning patients are mine to make."[5]

Practice Structure

Group and Staff Models

Medical staff organization will vary from plan to plan. Of fundamental importance is whether the model of the plan is group or staff. In a group model, physicians are organized into a professional group, which contracts with the HMO as an insurance entity. In this model, a highly developed staff structure can be expected. The group, in essence, belongs to the physicians. In such a structure there is generally a president of the medical staff and an executive body or committee. The group has a wide range of responsibilities that usually include physician compensation, benefits, hiring of new physicians, new services, expansion of the group, and negotiation and contracting—often on a global or capitation basis—for services provided by the medical group.

In some staff model HMOs, the organization takes on the appearance of an internal group, and may closely resemble a true group practice. There is usually a physician executive committee in place with representation from the full physician staff. A president of the group might be elected or the medical director may serve as chair of that body. Physician staff executive committees ultimately have less authority in a staff model HMO but are sure to be involved in approval of new clinical policies, participation in major decisions regarding expansion of services, approval of new physician members of the staff, and advancement of physicians. Both group and staff model organizations may impose a probationary or preliminary period prior to advancement to full or permanent status. Such status may or may not have implications regarding compensation for the physician under review.

In both group and staff model HMOs, a physician executive committee usually receives reports of committees and subcommittees and acts upon those requiring approval of the full physician group. In a staff model HMO, major policy decisions need to be approved by the board of the HMO. In a group model, the physician group acts with full authority in most matters, except for those that involve the insurance mechanism, which must be enacted within the decision-making process of the HMO. Liaison or linkage committees may function in these settings. In some staff model HMOs, the physicians are not organized into a grouplike structure; as such they would tend to relate more directly to the medical director or the president/CEO of the plan.

Salaries and Scheduling. As a rule, physicians who work in a staff or group model are salaried either by the HMO or the practice group. (Physicians who work with an IPA or network HMO generally are paid on a fee-for-service or a capitation basis, in which payment is a set dollar amount per month or year for each HMO member under their care.[6]) There are clearly variations on those arrangements, even within individual HMOs. Primary care HMO physicians typically work 28 to 36 hours a week of scheduled office time, but may possibly log up to 50 to 60 hours a week,[7] depending on on-call scheduling, hospital coverage, and the structure of the HMO. The average salary for primary care managed care physicians is competitive with primary care salaries in the private practice sector. As in the private practice (fee-for-service) sector, subspecialists in managed care continue to earn somewhat more than primary care physicians; however, the salary differential between specialists and primary care physicians is less in HMOs than in fee-for-service practice.

Team Medicine

Successful prepaid group practice depends upon effective teams and teamwork. Collegiality and teamwork are critical elements for success within any group practice.[8] Practicing within a medical team may present a challenge to some physicians. For the physician who has functioned completely alone in a solo practice setting, the change can be striking. Jack Silversin, DDS, MPH and Mary Jan Kornacki, MS, in describing the need for teamwork state, "While HMOs vary greatly in the way they are organized, managed and governed, they have in common the mission of providing the highest quality medical care for a fixed dollar. To do so requires a high level of communication and collaboration. And that needs . . . a high level of trust, subtlety and intimacy—in essence, teamwork."[9] Silversin and Kornacki go on to state,

> Physicians are trained and socialized into a profession that holds autonomy as a basic right. Many physicians join HMOs and other group practice settings believing that they can have the best of both worlds; that is, enjoy the advantages of being in a group and able to do things their own way. Physicians' value of autonomy affects not only their interactions with support staff, it may also undermine teamwork with professional colleagues. A lack of collaboration in these important relationships is likely to be a source of frustration when all physicians are busy and stress levels are high.[9]

Irving Klitsner, MD, one of the early physicians of the Southern California Permanente Medical Group notes,

> I was always uneasy about needing to take patients' economic histories to determine if they could afford my care. I was also attracted by the organizational structure and the objectives of Kaiser Permanente. From the beginning, this organization gave the physician responsibility for the quality of medical care and service. It also provided the challenge to develop and implement a new method of financing health care and to create a managed health care system that would be efficient and effective. Individuality is not stymied and innovation is encouraged.[10]

Practice Teams

Most staff or group model HMOs have practice teams made up of physicians, physician assistants, nurse practitioners, registered nurses, medical assistants, and receptionists. Success requires flexibility and adaptability on the part of all members of the team. Generally, each practice group of between four and ten physicians (often by area of specialty) designates a physician who assumes lead responsibilities. These responsibilities focus on providing services for the practice group's patient population. Often the physicians practice in single-specialty groups (family physicians working with family physicians, for example), but other arrangements exist in which multispecialty teams practice together, such as a family physician, pediatrician, and internist. The practice team may function in varied ways as well. In some organizations, each physician may practice fairly independently, with nursing support to manage the practice. In other organizations, the practice is set up so that a group of providers practices cohesively as a team.

In both situations, patients have primary care physicians who are responsible for helping to manage their care, but the nature of the cross-coverage and resultant responsibilities varies from practice to practice. Most HMOs use nurse practitioners and/or physician assistants quite extensively. In some instances, these professionals may serve as primary providers for a panel of patients, but more typically, nurse practitioners or physician assistants work with a physician or team of physicians to help care for a panel of patients. More specialized roles, such as nurse midwives, nurse practitioners, and physician assistants—who have more in-depth training in, for example, surgical or orthopedic diagnosis and treatment—are becoming more prevalent and enthusiastically endorsed by patients.

Nurses. Registered nurses (RNs) fulfill a number of invaluable roles in a staff or group model HMO. Coordination of the providers in the group is an essential role. RNs often provide telephone advice to patients who need information or support. Nurses may help staff specialty clinics and help assure continuity of patient care. Home care nurses and discharge planning nurses are indispensable in helping HMO physicians manage very sick outpatients while using the hospital efficiently. Licensed practical nurses (LPNs) and medical assistants support HMO physicians in much the same manner as in fee-for-service practice.

Primary Care Physicians As "Gatekeepers"

Much has been written about the "gatekeeper" role of physicians in HMOs. The primary care physician has been identified as a potential mechanism to solve two vexing issues in health care: excessive costs and excessive utilization. The premise of gatekeeping is that tighter control over utilization of services can be maintained by strategically placing the primary care physician in the role of manager of services, or "gatekeeper." From physicians' perspectives, this can be a sensitive issue as it places them in the role of advocate for both the patient and the organization. (For a more comprehensive discussion of the ethical issues arising from balancing cost with patient needs, see Chapter 3.) For example, because needs preside over wants in the managed care setting, some patients are likely to press physicians for services they perceive they need. HMO physicians, like all physicians, need to become skilled in directing their patients toward appropriate medical care. With demanding patients, this can be a challenge. A physician's interpersonal skills are therefore highly important, especially in the HMO setting.

Patient Encounters

Most patient encounters begin with a phone call. In most HMOs, the patient is preferably scheduled with his or her primary physician. When the primary physician is unavailable, one of his or her colleagues will see the patient. Most HMOs utilize provider schedules that are open for routine scheduled appointments, work-ins, and urgent care appointments. Other organizations have urgent care centers where physicians will see patients on an urgent basis and refer them back to their primary care physician for follow-up care. In either setting, the availability of the patient's medical record allows for rapid understanding of his or her ongoing problems and medications, as well as insight into interpersonal issues that may be important in facilitating a successful encounter. In most offices, after completion of the proper history and physical, lab work or X-rays may be obtained in the same building. Many HMOs have an on-site pharmacy if prescriptions are required. The dialogue between physician and pharmacist can help clarify a patient's case and help to assure a successful outcome for the patient.

Consultant Networks and Nonphysician Services

When a consultation with a specialist is needed, most HMOs have well-developed networks of consultants to whom a referral can be made. In most staff or group model HMOs, some of whose consultants are paid on a salary or capitation arrangement, there are fewer individual incentives to encourage referrals when indicated. In most HMOs, the consultant network is sufficiently developed so that a phone call to a consultant will often yield the requisite information. When a consultant is needed, arrangements are usually coordinated by the office staff. Appropriateness of consultation referral is monitored in staff or group model HMOs via peer review. Consultants are also subject to review.

Often, patients require care beyond the scope of that which a physician can deliver in the office. This care may best be delivered by nonphysicians who have a specific level of training and expertise in defined clinical areas. For example, home care nursing services, nutritional consultations, and health education services may be appropriate. HMOs have ready access to these services, an advantage that increases efficiency and quality of care. Most HMOs offer mental health services available by consultation. In many organizations, the mental health professionals work side-by-side with the physicians so that ready consultation is available for challenging cases.

On-Call Responsibilities

Staff model physicians can expect to be placed on call for urgent problems, typically once every fourth to eighth night. Patient coverage may include those belonging to one's own small team of practitioners or those of the entire practice. In general, there are many support services available to on-call physicians, such as a nurse triage function, wherein registered nurses handle calls concerning informational or relatively minor clinical decisions. The nurses then divert the more significant calls or questions to the on-call physician. Additional support may be available after-hours from either staff physicians or moonlighting physicians, who can handle urgent problems in the offices, obviating the need to refer patients to the emergency room. In addition to ambulatory on-call responsibilities, physicians are required to cover hospitalized patients as well.

Hospital Care

The culture at most HMOs views the hospital as an intervention. That is, hospitalization is a last resort, and home care services and other outpatient services are emphasized. Similar to non-HMO physicians, group practice HMO physicians are responsible for patient admissions, the rounding and routine daily care of patients, as well as the engagement of appropriate consultants. These arrangements may vary from organization to organization, and often from one team to another within the HMO. Many HMOs have developed shared rounding, where one physician in a team is responsible for managing hospital patients for a week at a time.

HMOs generally have continuing care nurses, RNs who assist the physician in assessing patient clinical needs. The continuing care nurse ensures that patient needs are met and facilitates patients' return home or to an alternative facility in as timely a fashion as possible. Physicians working with continuing care nurses often proactively preempt the hospital utilization review (UR) nurses' involvement in the care of the HMO's patients. In fact, in most HMOs the utilization review is conducted not as a separate function, but by the physicians themselves.

Guidelines for hospital care are typically provided to staff and group model HMO physicians. For IPA physicians, guidelines on hospital care are often subject to rules and incentives designed to influence their use of the hospital. Specific diagnoses require preauthorization for hospitalization or surgery in order to be covered by the IPA. Utilization review nurses in the IPA are available to assess the appropriateness of a patient's continuing stay in the hospital and to help arrange the necessary resources to facilitate a timely discharge.

Physician Roles and Responsibilities

All physicians are managers. Unlike physicians who practiced in the old-style fee-for-service setting, however, HMO clinicians consciously manage resources. HMO physicians, more than other physicians, must determine the proper use of technology, pharmaceuticals, nursing services, and time necessary to assess patient needs. They must also provide the best possible care for each patient. In this respect, each physician in an HMO setting must be a "gatekeeper."

Levels of responsibility for physicians vary from one HMO setting to another. In any setting, physicians usually have a number of responsibilities that extend beyond direct patient care. For example, the group as a whole typically undertakes the recruitment and orientation of physicians new to the HMO, coordination of vacation scheduling, continuing medical education (CME), staffing needs, and other key responsibilities. While all physicians are responsible for quality improvement and utilization management, a lead physician is usually responsible for ensuring that the group monitors the care they provide and that unnecessary variation is minimized. All physicians are increasingly expected to analyze data, such as profiles of physician practice patterns. Similarly, physician groups are developing and implementing local clinical guidelines, a process in which the individual physician can expect to participate.

Departments

Each physician, whether primary care or specialized, will be a member of a department. Physicians may be grouped according to specialty. In other settings, physicians work out of smaller or multidisciplinary offices. Departments serve purposes such as:

- fostering collegiality and interaction among physicians
- fostering the development of clinical guidelines and standards; for example, well-child guidelines developed by a department of pediatrics
- sharing developed guidelines with other departments interested in those clinical services
- promoting discussion and assessment of new services and developments within the HMO that may affect the clinical work of the department; for example, hospital rounding, changes in hospital policies, regulatory developments, and new innovations

Committees

All HMOs, like hospital staffs and large medical groups, depend on a wide array of committees to carry out their objectives. Some committees are mandated by regulatory bodies, others are formed by the HMO, and some are formed as task forces. Some committees generally found within HMOs are:

- Quality Assurance
- Utilization Management/Utilization Review
- Health Education
- Health Promotion
- CME/Library/Physician Education
- Medical Records
- Safety
- Morbidity and Mortality

In summary, a group or staff model practice has many inherent strengths. First, there is the sharing of essential patient information through use of a uniform medical record. This facilitates a flow of information from physician to physician and other providers that greatly enhances the quality of information exchanged and, potentially, the quality of care delivered. Multidisciplinary collaboration for shared patients has significant advantages when dealing with the most challenging clinical cases. Usually, a case conference can readily be called, and serves the dual purpose of enhancing patient management as well as efficiency (eliminating redundancy) and quality of care. Finally, with managed care setting the pace for health care's transformation to quality management, group practices are finding exciting new applications of quality improvement techniques for enhanced process and outcome of patient care (see Chapters 6 and 8).

AVOIDING BURNOUT: OPTIONS FOR CAREER REVITALIZATION

Over the long haul, any career can lose its original luster, and the practice of medicine is no exception. Regardless of practice setting, physicians—particularly those in primary care—are prone to burnout. It is no secret that many physicians today are dissatisfied with the current climate of increased regulation, scrutiny of performance, and competition for patients. You may one day consider a career shift or even wish to leave medical practice. Early intervention is the key to preventing burnout. We must be proactive in finding ways to challenge and rejuvenate ourselves and our careers.

New Skills Development

New skills development can revitalize our work lives. Fortunately, the regular and flexible hours in HMO practice afford physicians the luxury of time to pursue other interests, both personal and professional. A newfound sense of satisfaction can be found in learning to perform a new procedure, such as flexible sigmoidoscopy, cardiac stress testing, or an ear, nose, and throat examination. Some physicians, however, may find the need to redirect their careers. Managed care physicians have the advantage of being able to choose from a variety of career opportunities. While many physicians choose to devote themselves exclusively to patient care, others seek participation in and contribution to the larger organization through committee work, improvement projects, and self-development. Some may even wish to develop a new specialty, such as medical orthopedics, geriatrics, nursing home care, urgent care, or hospital-based care, among other potential avenues.

Teaching Opportunities

Beyond medically related changes or additions to practice are shifts in direction that may take the physician away from clinical activity. For example, as a high proportion of HMOs are affiliated with academic institutions and hospitals, and are sometimes full medical school affiliates, teaching opportunities for managed care physicians are burgeoning. The current national push for primary care education and teaching within ambulatory sites has led to combined efforts between these two worlds. Ambulatory settings provide excellent opportunities for new physicians to gain hands-on experience in the essentials of HMO practice, including preventive and ambulatory care, home care, and telephone advice. These settings also orient the new physician to the foundations of quality improvement and utilization management.

Resident Training Programs

The Kaiser organizations in California, Group Health Cooperative of Puget Sound, in Washington, and Long Island Jewish Hospital in New York offer on-site residency training programs. Two other programs that typify this cooperative spirit are the primary care internal medicine residency programs of Harvard Community Health Plan in Boston, Massachusetts, and Health Care Plan in Buffalo, New York. Harvard Community Health Plan, with Brigham and Women's Hospital, created an internal medicine residency program based partly in the hospital and partly in ambulatory sites of Harvard Community Health Plan.[11] Health Care Plan developed a similar program at the same time with the department of internal medicine of the State University of New York at Buffalo. In this program, a resident is paired with an attending physician/mentor who serves as a practice partner for the resident during the full three years of the residency training program.

Medical Management Careers

Many may view management responsibilities within the HMO as a natural extension of one's existing charges, as HMOs tend to foster a mix of clinical practice with medical management. As management activities expand, clinical effort tends to recede. As a general rule, retaining clinical involvement is essential to maintaining clinician credibility among physician colleagues. Nonetheless, physicians are needed more than ever in management roles. Programs offering continuing education are growing (see Chapter 4), and board certification in medical management is a near reality. The HMO Group, an alliance of 18 HMOs from around the country, is one such group dedicated to furthering the education of managed care physicians through conferences and seminars. The HMO Group sponsors *HMO Practice*, a national, peer-reviewed medical journal devoted to the needs of physicians in managed care.

Research Opportunities

Research is yet another growth area for HMO physicians. With their large populations, HMOs represent an enormous potential resource for health services research. A number of larger and well-established HMOs such as Group Health Cooperative of Puget Sound in Washington and Kaiser Permanente in Portland, Oregon, and Oakland, California have well-developed, outstanding research programs. Research opportunities, however, do not exist only at the macro level. Quality improvement methodology utilizes health services research techniques and is serving as a stimulus to further research efforts in all HMOs. Collaboration between HMOs and academic and research entities is likely to proliferate in order to meet the demand for physicians trained in research design and methodology.

Population-based research responds in part to initiatives from external granting sources. For example, Group Health Cooperative of Puget Sound has studied the efficacy of bike helmets in preventing head injury among bicyclists and fall prevention among the elderly, and has also co-sponsored the landmark Rand Health Insurance Experiment. Kaiser Permanente Medical Care Program in Oakland, California, reviewed the epidemiology of ulcerative colitis and Crohn's disease and the long-term reduction of colon cancer, attributable to the application of sigmoidoscopy. These projects represent the kind of action-oriented research in which HMOs excel.

The second kind of research is allied with quality management. Data are gathered as part of a diagnostic journey and conclusions are reached based on the analysis of the data. This type of research can be highly practical and specific to the needs of HMOs, and typically focuses on outcomes research, utilization management, technology management, and quality improvement. Examples are appropriate use of prostate-specific antigen; patient preferences in prostate and breast surgery;[12] and physician/practice behavior change regarding influenza vaccination. The Upstate HMO Research and Education Collaborative was created as a joint venture of the three group practice HMOs of upstate New York: Community Health Plan in Albany, Health Services Medical Corporation in Syracuse, and Health Care Plan in Buffalo. The combined plans bring together a population base of over 350,000 members.

This is by no means a comprehensive list of nonclinical career options for managed care physicians. The demand for practitioners in utilization management, quality management, involvement in educational programs, and community leadership positions, among others, is expected to grow.

CONCLUSION

The debate over whether prepaid group practice indeed reduces cost and provides patient care superior to traditional fee-for-service will predictably continue unabated for some time to come. What is not debated, however, is the fact that managed care is a viable practice alternative to traditional fee-for-service practice. There are many pluses to a career in managed care. Some choose it for pragmatic reasons—reasonable hours, a comfortable income, its

---

Exhibit 2–1 The Ideal Practice

> In the prepaid group practice there is potential to achieve the ideal practice pattern. Features of prepaid group practice that can promote the ideal include the opportunity to:
> — develop physician-patient relationships uncontaminated by any financial negotiation or barrier.
> — compete with other physicians in the realm of professional excellence rather than economics.
> — accomplish clinical research with a defined population.
> — teach and disseminate health information to a large member population and influence them regarding reasonable health care expectations.
> — share patient care issues and knowledge with colleagues through conferences and rounds facilitated by common medical records.
> — enjoy job security and tenure.
> — take pride in being associated with highly skilled and respected physicians.
> — develop new skills or subspecialty interests, including physician management.
> — practice quality and ethical medicine in a quasi-academic environment.
> — teach students and residents.
> — access formal and informal consultations.
> — be free from running the business of medical practice.
> — plan and schedule a reasonable life-style.
>
> There are also aspects of prepaid group practice that present challenges to the physician striving to develop the ideal practice. To meet these challenges, physicians must:
> — be motivated and productive without the fee-for-service monetary incentive.
> — satisfy patients who seek care with a sense of entitlement to services.
> — balance cost containment activities and quality of care, regardless of income concerns.
> — accept a reputation and status that is judged by the caliber of the department or group rather than the individual.
> — be receptive to colleagues and administrators offering advice or even criticism.
> — develop a sense of ownership and pride in the organization.
>
> *Source*: Reprinted from Klitsner I, The pediatrician in the HMO, in *HMO Practice*, Vol 4:6, pp. 206–208, with permission of *HMO Practice*, © 1990.

rational approach to on-call and hospital coverage, or avoidance of the business side of medical practice. Others choose this path for the idealism on which the movement was founded, and wish to be part of a "new wave." (See Exhibit 2–1.) Such physicians find HMOs a highly attractive choice that is likely to meet their idealistic expectations. These individuals are inclined to place a premium on solid outcomes information, preventive services, the ideal of maximizing patient access to services, and continuous quality improvement.

Among adherents of managed care, the current atmosphere is one of renewed energy and commitment. There is a growing sense among HMOs that the original values that led to the creation of prepaid group practice are now being fulfilled. In Exhibit 2–1, Irving Klitsner, one of the pioneers of prepaid group practice, presents his views on the ideal HMO practice and the challenges that lie ahead. As we move into the future, quality improvement, team practice, outcomes research, and patient-centered care will become fully integrated into the practice of medicine. In the authors' opinion, both the challenges and opportunities that await the profession are exciting and welcome.

REFERENCES

1. Nelson JA. The history and spirit of the HMO movement: the early years. *HMO Practice*. 1987;1:75–85.
2. Relman A. Reforming the health care system. *N Engl J Med*. 1990;323:991–992.
3. Wennberg JE. A challenge to HMOs. *HMO Practice*. 1992;6:5–10.
4. Jacobs L. Making the change. *HMO Practice*. 1990;4:215–219.
5. Sheehan TP. The family practitioner in the HMO. *HMO Practice*. 1990;4:209–210.
6. Hillman AL. Financial incentives for physicians in HMOs: is there a conflict of interest? *N Engl J Med*. 1987;317:1743-1748.
7. James T III, Nash DB. Health maintenance organizations: a new development or the emperor's new clothes? In: Nash DB, ed. *Future Practice Alternatives in Medicine*. 2nd ed. New York, NY: Igaku-Shoin Medical Publishers; 1993.
8. Friedson E. *Doctoring together: a study of professional social control*. Chicago, Ill.: The University of Chicago Press;1975.
9. Silversin J, Kornacki MJ. The HMO physician as team player. *HMO Practice*. 1990;4:226–230.
10. Klitsner I. The pediatrician in the HMO. *HMO Practice*. 1990;4:206–208.
11. Epstein AL, Pollack DK. The HMO and the academic medical center: a primary care residency. *HMO Practice*. 1988;2:133-138.
12. Wennberg J. Outcomes research, cost containment, and the fear of health care rationing. *N Engl J Med*. 1990;323:1202–1204.

Editorial Commentary

Susan L. Howell
David B. Nash

For those who want to know what practicing in an HMO environment is really like, physicians Leonard A. Katz and Michael W. Cropp are the right people to ask. Dr. Katz is current editor of *HMO Practice* and is a senior clinician at a large staff model HMO in Buffalo, New York and a full-time faculty member at the University of Buffalo Medical School. Dr. Cropp, a family physician in Buffalo, also practices in a staff model HMO.

The authors provide the reader with a look at life in an HMO practice from an "in the trenches" perspective. They examine such issues as the mechanics and structure of HMO practice, workload, opportunities for advancement, academic enhancement, practice expectations among the various HMO models, and the professional characteristics that typify the managed care physician. (Complementing Dr. Katz's and Dr. Cropp's chapter is Chapter 4 on the role of the physician manager.)

The authors portray the perceived pros and cons of working in the managed care setting. A structured practice environment, potential to take on nonclinical responsibilities, considerable freedom from administrative responsibility (i.e., the numbing degree of paperwork often associated with fee-for-service practice), and the satisfaction of helping patients to stay well over the long run are among managed care's numerous attractions. Because of its stability and regular hours, a managed care practice affords a viable way to combine one's career, family, and personal life. No longer need physicians concede that career and family are, by virtue of the demands of the profession, mutually exclusive.

The authors also address employee burnout, loss of autonomy, and some of the inevitable strains imposed on the physician in the gatekeeper role. They acknowledge that while an HMO practice may not be for everyone, it offers challenges and rewards heretofore unimagined by the profession. No longer a great experiment, managed care is here to stay. The authors invite you to glimpse a future that could be right for you.

Chapter 3

Ethical Issues in Managed Care and Managed Competition: Problems and Promises

John La Puma
David Schiedermayer

INTRODUCTION

Medicine is a moral enterprise, and managed care organizations (MCOs), because they are involved in the delivery of medical care, are moral entities. Managed care (and managed competition) also recognize their inherent economic tenets. Managed care's goals of quality health care delivery, cost containment, and equality of access demand that physicians be both patient advocate and organizational advocate, even when these roles seem to conflict. A re-emphasis of managed care's moral mission is essential in enabling physicians, patients, payers, and policymakers to fulfill their new roles, and to preserve the fidelity of the doctor-patient relationship.

In this chapter, we attempt to illustrate how physicians can maintain a high standard of ethical and compassionate care in the MCO setting. Although valid technical, organizational, and financial distinctions exist between HMOs, PPOs, and IPAs, we do not try to elucidate these distinctions. Just as physicians of many different specialties find common ground in the relationships that make medicine worth practicing, the various forms of MCOs share common goals and ideals. Managed competition is also undergirded by similar key ethical assumptions. We define these terms and delineate these assumptions. Using case studies, we review the benefits and burdens of managed care. We examine potential changes in managed care under the Clinton administration. Finally, we grapple with the sorts of issues patients, physicians, and payers might expect to confront in their roles as professionals in the managed care field.

31

MANAGED CARE: DEFINITIONS

Managed care organizations are intended to prevent disease,[1] promote health, and provide access to care more equitably and affordably than under fee-for-service practice.[2] The Institute of Medicine's Committee on Utilization Management by Third Parties defines managed care as "a set of techniques used by or on behalf of purchasers of health care benefits . . . (to influence) patient care decision making through case-by-case assessments of the appropriateness of care."[1] Its essential features are restricted choice of provider; an extensive peer review system; negotiated prices and risk sharing arrangements with physicians; responsibility for a defined population; and integration of insurance and direct provision of services under a fixed prospective budget.[3]

More than 34 million Americans now receive medical care managed through HMOs, PPOs, or external review organizations. Managed care enrollments are growing; most insurers will use managed care methods in the move toward the managed competition systems of the future.

Managed care systems share a general philosophy of care that prizes appropriateness, necessity, and cost-effectiveness.[4-8] Managed care systems that strive to insure patients, diffuse financial risks, deliver health services, and maintain personal patient satisfaction will be the model health care systems of the 1990s.

Many MCOs monitor practice by using programs in quality assurance and utilization management; by contracting with regional referral facilities for high technology, high-cost procedures, and by holding individual physicians accountable for the amount of money they authorize ("spend") per enrollee per month. Case management is used to effect cost savings, especially in long-term care. MCOs are actively engaged in the analysis of health care quality and clinical outcomes (from patient satisfaction to technology assessment) to provide better service and contain costs.

The ethical assumptions of managed care will shape medical practice in the coming years. Managed care and managed competition recognize the dual concepts of appropriateness and scarcity: if all care were of high quality and appropriate,[9] and if resources were unlimited, managed care would be unnecessary. Managed care requires primary physicians to be resource agents, and assumes that physicians will be both patient and MCO advocates, even when these roles seem to conflict. British generalists perform both roles implicitly, and invoke medical reasons to deny medical treatment to patients "too old, too sick, or too unlikely to benefit."[10,11] Patients generally are not told that the resource is relatively scarce.

Although managed care methods are touted to reduce costs and ensure quality, and are featured in most health care reform packages, reports exist of patient dissatisfaction;[12–15] financial conflicts in decision making;[16–18] physician discontent with MCOs and the gatekeeper role;[19–22] legal challenges to MCO review and reviewer authority;[23,24] and mixed cost and quality effects.[1,25]

THE ETHICAL ASSUMPTIONS OF MANAGED CARE

Managed care organizations (MCOs) are founded on at least three ethical assumptions: equality of access is the proper ethical concept for resolving allocation dilemmas; the doctor-patient relationship will be fiduciary and nonadversarial; and quality assurance and utilization management will be confidential and effective.

- **Equality of access** for all MCO members is more important than the option of all-out, expensive treatment for one member. This concept of equality requires that MCO physicians be consistent decision makers, making the same decisions for individual patients as for groups of comparable patients.
- Managed care also relies on the principle that **doctor-patient relationships will be trusting and covenantal,** even when contractually based. Physicians will act with goodwill and will be patient advocates, e.g., when appropriate, they will appeal economic constraints on an individual patient's care. Accordingly, patients will trust their physicians to work with them within the system.
- Managed care is undergirded by the ethical precept that **quality assurance activities and utilization management func-**

tions will be educational and confidential, and will be used to promote quality care rather than to punish patients or physicians.

Traditionally, the goals of managed care have been to improve access, prevent disease, promote health, and contain costs. MCO goals, however, should not focus simply on controlling providers' practices and containing costs. Without attention to its ethical underpinnings, managed care may not resolve policy dilemmas of justice, may adversely affect quality, and may not reduce costs in the long run.[26]

The ethical constraints in managed care result in specific benefits and burdens to all parties in the relationship.

Benefits to Patients

The benefits to patients in MCOs are substantial. Although MCOs differ in structure and function,[27] the philosophy of managed care discourages overtreatment, encourages general preventive care, and attempts to promote both cost containment and quality health care delivery. MCOs integrate the financing and delivery of health services, provide services at a discount, and minimize paperwork. Copayments and deductibles are low or nonexistent. In one study, the quality and quantity of ambulatory care for HMO patients was judged equal to or better than that of fee-for-service patients.[28]

Benefits to Physicians

MCOs are also beneficial to physicians. MCOs limit practice start-up costs and many MCOs offer dependable incomes, regular practice hours, and structured practices.[29] MCOs also review and validate physician credentials, setting a minimum standard of practice for their organizations.[30] MCOs give physicians financial incentives to deliver care in an efficient, cost-effective manner. Physicians are also assured a patient population, albeit at volume discount.

Benefits to Payers

MCOs offer equal access for all members, provide financial reimbursement for administrators and others, and allow payers to use developed business principles and test those priniciples in new markets. For example, the principles of continuous quality improvement have been used in the auto industry since the 1970s and are now being applied by some MCOs to the administration of health care.[9,31,32]

Burdens to Patients

There are burdens for managed care patients. Given medicine's traditional focus on the individual patient, MCO emphasis on group benefit may seem utilitarian and even impersonal. Some patients receive incomplete or incomprehensible information when an MCO plan is offered or advertised.[33] Restrictions on care are de-emphasized, and patients must at least consider scrutinizing both payer and physician. Patients may no longer be able to trust the physician to have their best interests at heart, as physicians no longer serve just one master. These and other practical questions arise about patient autonomy,[34,35] and patients' ability to access particular providers and services that may not be covered by their MCO plan.

Burdens to Physicians

Managed care presents moral and professional challenges to medicine's virtue-based ethics, including the fundamental values and assumed prerogatives of clinical practice.[36] Managed care's administrative controls may change doctor-patient relationships to businessperson-consumer relationships.[37,38] The administrative complexity and standardization of MCO processes do not easily accommodate differences between individual patients, stifling flexibility.[39] The physician is increasingly caught between patient expectations of more and higher-tech care and the MCO's expectations of cost containment.

Burdens to Payers

MCOs are often financially risky enterprises; they are responsible for an enormous array of services. Health care expenditures are often perversely unresponsive to rational administrative techniques. MCOs also suffer from a dearth of outcome data, and are often unable to substantiate their protocols and procedures with valid, reliable medical data. MCOs may be liable in many situations. Areas of liability include breach of contract, breach of warranty, breach of the implied covenant of good faith and fair dealing, and breach of the relationship between patient and physician. In addition, payers are subject to litigation concerning price fixing, fee or compensation arrangements, and monopolization. Finally, payers are responsible for attracting and credentialing credible, respected clinicians as reviewers, heightening administrative and professional regulation.[40]

CASES IN CONFLICT: ETHICS CONSULTATION IN THE MCO

The role of ethics consultations in the MCO setting can help clarify the ethical assumptions in managed care and avoid unfair burdens on any one party. The ethics consultation in a particular patient's case can be the first step in resolving conflicts of interests and in generating new institutional responses to issues. MCOs may wish to employ ethics consultants in the future; ethics consultation would be part of the benefits package offered by the MCO to those who enroll. Ethics consultants are professionals with specialized training and expertise that equips them to identify, analyze, and help resolve moral problems that arise in patient care. A consultant should personally deal with the patient. A consultant should possess clinical judgment; communicate effectively with the health care team members; negotiate and facilitate negotiations; and teach others how to analyze and resolve similar problems in similar cases.[41]

Sometimes ethics consultation involves determining when a physician might have to assume the role of patient financial advocate. For example, corporate profit-sharing plans, including some physician-hospital joint ventures,[42] can threaten to pit the economic interest of the physician against the economic and treatment interests of patients. But MCO physicians do have the new duty of explicit financial advocacy,[43] as MCO disclosure to patients may be insufficient to enable them to make informed choices about care.[44] Prior to the advent of MCOs, the physician attempted to hospitalize medically indigent patients by quietly managing the admissions system. Now, when a patient needs hospital care, the physician must make an explicit clinical case with the guardians of the MCO budget.

When conflicts of interest are present, the patient or proxy should be informed. While such disclosure may be insufficient, an ethics consultant may teach negotiation strategy to colleagues. Physicians have to know the MCO well enough to make patients and their families aware of financial constraints so they can search for alternative funding, rearrange personal assets, or appeal the constraints directly. Patients denied access for financial reasons to medically indicated treatment should not be led to believe the denial is for medical reasons. Explicit financial information is necessary for patients and their families to make fully informed choices about alternative medical treatments. The federal requirements that emergency patients be informed when transferred for financial reasons illustrate this new aspect of informed consent.[45,46,47,48]

The doctor-patient-MCO relationship requires that physicians enforce the organization's own moral responsibilities of facilitating members' access to health care and handling confidential information carefully.[49] Physicians can help design systems of managed care that permit ethical practice overall;[50] even so, unfair constraints may occur in individual cases. In the past, physicians have successfully appealed constraints on out-of-plan services.[47,51] Appealing these constraints is a newly explicit burden, one that is likely to become more commonplace.[52] Whether doctors will continue to help patients appeal these constraints will depend in part on the strength and depth of their relationships, and on the effect of constraints on the quality of care.

Equality of Access — Case Examples

MCOs require doctors to provide all members with equal access to the MCO's medical resources, and still prescribe care on the basis of an individual member's medical needs.

MCOs depend on physicians to protect the financial well-being of the MCO and to be mindful of the medical and financial interests of all MCO members. Most MCOs could ill afford to provide all the medical care needed for persistent vegetative state patients, no matter how vocal their proxies.[53] For MCOs, equality of access means that if one patient's needs are huge, meeting those needs makes meeting the needs of other patients much more financially difficult. To provide basic care to all members, certain expensive benefits, such as liver or bone marrow transplantation, are often excluded from MCO care.

The primary obligation of most physicians is still the health of an individual patient, rather than the medical and financial well-being of all MCO members, or the MCO itself.[54] To meet MCO expectations, some physicians may be obliged to limit the care given to a specially medically needy patient so that scarce resources will be available to other patients.[55] Indigent MCO patients may, for example, receive fewer resources than nonindigent MCO patients. They may also have a higher prevalence of serious symptoms and more hospital bed-days than other non-MCO patients.[56]

To increase the appropriateness of care, and provide equal access to care having reasonable efficacy, few untoward effects, and low costs, MCOs advocate the standardization of clinical protocols for the individual physician.[57] Patients and doctors, however, view clinical medicine as an effort of particularities. Physicians who treat both managed care and fee-for-service patients may use different rationales for determining whether to refer patients for procedures or desired services: whether MCO patients actually receive fewer services than patients with indemnity insurance is debated.[9,58] The referral issue can arise in both high technology medicine and everyday office practice, as the following cases demonstrate. These cases also demonstrate that the ethical issues in managed care are often common and universal and are also found in fee-for-service care. The ethical practice of MCO medicine is similar in many ways to the ethical practice of medicine in other systems. Ethical issues in managed care, however, seem to focus more directly on access and cost, because these aspects are more explicitly imbedded in the organizational structure of the MCO system.

Case 1. Fern Mead is a 17-year-old female who comes to the office complaining of recurrent acne. She was seen two weeks ago for the same problem. Ms. Mead is running for high school homecoming queen, and is concerned that her medical condition will interfere with her popularity and candidacy. In addition, she has a new boyfriend, and he won't kiss her unless her face gets better. She has tried topical clindamycin, benzoyl peroxide 10% lotion, and oral doxycycline every day for two weeks. She now wants to see a dermatologist.

Examination reveals a pleasant, shy young woman in no acute distress. She is afebrile. There are no cystic lesions on the face, neck, shoulders, or back. Some scarring and pitting is present over the face, however, and active comedones are present in various stages of healing. There is mild improvement from two weeks ago.

The ethics consultant in this case happens to be the primary physician, and knows well the managed care organization's rules regarding specialist referral. Patients are not to be referred unless there is cystic acne or the disease is unresponsive to conventional treatment. Should the physician follow the reasonable request of a patient with a medically minor, but psychologically and socially important condition and attempt to advocate for her (uncovered) treatment? To do so, the physician must either break the rules of the MCO by gaming the system or make a special effort to get the requested referral covered. Or should the physician protect his or her own pocketbook and endorse either the MCO rules, or the patient's attempt at advocacy—likely to be less effective than the physician's? Or should the physician ask the patient to pay for the referral herself?

The physician persuaded Ms. Mead to continue on her present course, promising to refer her if more improvement was not evidenced in ten days, at a return visit.

The patient continued her medication, improving a little more, but not substantially. In a return visit, the physician completed the consultation referral form for two visits to the dermatologist; the form arrived at the patient's home by mail nine days later. The dermatologist saw Ms. Mead within the next week, and prescribed a different antibiotic, facial soap, and lotion. She improved with several return visits, encouragement, and an additional referral.

In MCOs, physicians may be encouraged to act like vendors of a limited service; patients may then begin to act like customers competing for limited goods. Under these circumstances, patients can become demanding, and physicians can come to regard them as troublesome buyers. Patients may finally regard physicians as obstructive bureaucratic clerks who "owe" them already purchased products: examinations, prescriptions, referrals, and procedures.

Case 2. John Vandehey, a 55-year-old male, was admitted to the hospital with gastrointestinal bleeding and liver failure. Further evaluation revealed a primary hepatic carcinoma of fibrolamellar type. Mr. Vandehey was employed and belonged to an HMO. The transplant service was willing to perform a liver transplant and with the patient's consent, listed the patient as awaiting a suitable donor organ. The HMO said it would not pay for the expensive therapy it termed *experimental*. The patient's HMO internist called the ethics consultant after unsuccessfully appealing the HMO ruling to its medical director. "What do you think about the ethics of the refusal to permit the surgery?" she asked the consultant.

In this case, in contrast to case 1, the high technology nature of the consultation and procedure required the immediate outlay of significant financial resources. What is the obligation of MCOs to pay for innovative therapy? Was the MCO position arbitrary, or clearly spelled out in the patient's contract? What is the extent of the duty of a physician-gatekeeper to control costs for the health care corporation? Does this duty consist of merely informing the patient of the heretofore unknown financial constraint, or does it consist of appealing the constraint or directing the patient to alternative sources of legal or financial assistance? How does the physician address the relationship between his or her own salary and the profitability of the HMO? The growing literature that addresses these questions were discussed and debated in the process of the consultation.[59-64]

The ethics consultant assisted the physician and Mr. Vandehey in locating alternative funding from a state-supported fund for experimental therapy. While the search for other resources was underway, the patient was readmitted with abdominal pain, melena, and coagulopathy. An emergency liver transplant was attempted, but was unsuccessful; Mr. Vandehey died on the operating table.

In this case, the MCO's decision not to fund the transplant was, in retrospect, a reasonable one. In hospital-based treatment, the patient's viewpoint is often the expectation of unlimited access to higher technology care. Patients often expect that any care that is remotely likely to have a medical benefit will be offered.[65] Patients often do not expect that their doctors will limit care based on other patients' medical or financial considerations. They also may not expect the MCO to ration beneficial services for which they have paid, albeit as part of a group.[66] As long as the current professional and public fascination with expensive high technology continues, the intermediary role will be uncomfortable for physicians, who must either struggle to advocate financially for a patient or explain to a patient that access to a therapy is denied because it will cost other MCO members too much money.

The Doctor-Patient Relationship: Case Examples

The nature of the MCO doctor-patient relationship is not ethically distinct from doctor-patient relationships in indemnity systems. It is still a fiduciary relationship. The doctor still treats patients one at a time as unique and valued individuals; the doctor is still a prudent steward wisely judging the limits of care.

To be effective patient advocates, doctors must help patients balance medical benefits and financial risks. In a sense, MCO physicians are responsible for helping patients achieve this balance. Patients presently seek MCO contracts under a wide variety of situations: when healthy or ill, of their own free will or under duress, as a good financial decision, or under financial inducement or constraint.[67-69] Often, patients may not understand their medical conditions well enough to request or accept the care they may need.[70,71] The following case demonstrates the therapeutic value of good communication with patients. A positive case out-come should sometimes be enhanced trust, enabled by the human touch instead of increased treatment.[72]

Case 3. Arlene Cass is a 43-year-old mother of two with multi-ple sclerosis, admitted with an aspiration pneumonia. Her hus-band is on the faculty of the medical school and both are enrolled in the institution's IPA. After three days of treatment the patient is improved enough to converse and refuse antibiotics and tube feeding. The ethics consultant, also a member of the IPA, was asked if this refusal should be permitted. On examination, the patient says she does not wish to die, but she fears choking on her food, and says, "I don't want to end up like my uncle," who had severe Alzheimer's disease and was unable to make decisions.

The consultant met with Mrs. Cass's husband, 22-year-old daughter, and 17-year-old son. The patient's husband says that his wife is intellectually and physically frustrated. The husband wants her to accept tube feeding, believing that she is slightly confused and does not know her own mind. The patient, howev-er, says she does and wants to make her own decisions, saying, "I trust no one."

On exam she is alert but has obvious atrophy and severe skele-tal deformities. She has a 5-centimeter stage III sacral pressure sore, active bowel sounds, and a nontender abdomen. Her speech is slow and languorous. Her affect is sad, her mood unhappy, and her recent memory good. The patient is unable to move any of her extremities except her right arm.

The consultant found that the patient had partial decision-mak-ing capacity. Although it was costly to the IPA to continue her treatment, the consultant recommended that her decision be respected, and that increased personal and intellectual stimula-tion be afforded her. He specifically suggested tape-recorded books. The patient decided to accept antibiotics and a feeding tube as long as she was mentally alert.

In the end, the patient left the hospital without a feeding tube. She thanked the consultant for seeing her and listening to her intellectual agenda.

Most physicians and patients want to have trusting, mutually rewarding relationships. As recently as a decade ago, most doctors and patients knew what was expected: the doctor acted in the patient's best interests, managed the case, and held in confidence all information learned from or about the patient.[73,74] The patient trusted the doctor, did his or her best to get better, and told the truth.

Unfortunately, in managed care, role confusion is not uncommon for both doctors and patients.[75,76] A new contractual ethos can fit poorly within the established doctor-patient relationship norms of fidelity and honesty.[77] MCOs have strong incentives to discover "confidential" information, such HIV status, for example. MCO interviews with patients may subjugate informed consent, overtly breach confidentiality,[78] and reveal more concern for limiting care than providing it.[79] The working doctor-patient relationship is sometimes transformed into a dysfunctional doctor-patient-MCO ménage à trois.[80,81] Instead of a covenantal medical ethic based on trust, MCOs can rely on wariness,[82] accountability, and documentation; they have sometimes forced a reconsideration of fidelity, and endorsed a colder, more contractual medicolegal ethic.

Case 4. Frank O'Leary was 56 years old and a 30-year veteran of a major metropolitan police force. Mr. O'Leary had intractable pain from widespread metastatic prostate cancer to bone and bone marrow. While visiting his doctor in his MCO, he fell in the hallway, and sustained subdural and subarachnoid hematomas. A computed tomographic (CT) scan showed the hematomas, but the neurosurgeon did not find the patient to be a surgical candidate because of his prostate cancer and overall condition. The patient was transferred to the ICU, however, where he was ventilator-dependent and unresponsive. The patient's family was furious and blamed the nurses in the health plan's clinic for permitting the patient to fall. His wife threatened a lawsuit, saying, "I am hostile. I am not paying for death—the city is. He is a fighter and it does not matter if he feels a little pain. A little pain will not hurt him." She wanted to know why he wasn't getting more aggressive treatment for his cancer—was the MCO trying to save money on him even now?

The ethics consultant was called to negotiate with the family about their disagreements with his MCO care. On exam, the patient was unresponsive, intubated, febrile, tachycardic, and lacked spontaneous respiratory efforts. He had absent doll's eyes and corneals, although he withdrew both feet to pain. He had flaccid extremities and positive Babinskis bilaterally. He had a platelet count of 12,000.

The consultant found that Mr. O'Leary had not given any advance directives on life-sustaining treatment. He suggested that emergency cardiopulmonary resuscitation (CPR) was contraindicated because of the presence of rib metastases. Although the patient's wife was a reliable proxy decision maker, the consultant believed that further medical treatment was likely to be futile and suggested a brain scan and clergy support to the family to ameliorate their anger. He also suggested a brain flow scan.

The patient started breathing spontaneously, so no brain flow scan was ordered. Pastoral support was helpful. An MCO nurse spoke at length with the family, reassuring them that the patient was receiving good intensive care, and that an electroencephalogram (EEG) showed little brain activity. Upon hearing this, Mrs. O'Leary assented to a do not resuscitate (DNR) order.

The patient died in the intensive care unit (ICU) on the ventilator one week later; CPR was not performed.

This case illustrates the importance of sensitive communication even in the setting of a disgruntled family member or a threatened lawsuit. The MCO's nurse turned the case around, and the ethics consultant counseled against futile CPR simply for appearance's sake or to appease the patient's wife. The next two cases also illustrate the importance of retaining a good doctor-patient relationship in the MCO setting.

Case 5. Bruce Lindquist, 49, was chronically ill, severely retarded, dependent on Medicare and Medicaid, and enrolled in a state-sponsored MCO. Mr. Lindquist was successfully treated for urosepsis in the hospital. He had not required hospitalization in the past two years. During that time, he lived in a nursing home where he was spoon-fed by his mother and nurse's aides. After several days of intravenous antibiotics, the patient was no longer acutely ill, but continued to refuse oral feeding. A nasogastric tube was inserted and an ethics consultation was requested to evaluate the appropriateness of withdrawing tube feeding.

The consultation request did not suggest a financial foundation for the consultation, but rather assistance in evaluating the ethical issues of the burdens and benefits of tube feeding and clinical decision making for incompetent patients. Privately, however, the intern told the ethics consultant, "The problem is that this patient is a drain on society. How much longer can society afford it?"

The ethics consultant examined Mr. Lindquist and spoke with his mother and the house officers. Although his mother was concerned about procedures that might cause him to suffer, she felt that tube feeding would be beneficial, at least to see if he could regain his strength and appetite. Some house officers expressed discomfort with explicitly considering financial matters at the bedside, but others felt it to be an important part of the patient's care. The consultant advised that tube feeding should be continued and that the patient be placed in a new nursing home capable of providing this treatment. After several weeks of convalescence, Mr. Lindquist again began to take food by mouth and was able to return to his former nursing home and his mother's care.

In Mr. Lindquist's case, it was a perceived pressure to conserve public funds that suggested consideration of withdrawal of potentially life-sustaining therapy. The MCO was not involved in this consideration per se. But even if the MCO put constraints on the care, and even if financial constraints resulted in a change in clinical management, ethical care may not necessarily have been breached. For example, there may be no clear medical duty to provide elective, cosmetic procedures. When MCO or external financial constraints may directly result in injury, death, or disability, however, the physician's duty as a patient advocate is more clearly summoned.

Case 6. Carl Schmidt was a 54-year-old male found unresponsive at home and subsequently hospitalized. He had been employed and self-sufficient until two months prior to admission. Mr. Schmidt was enrolled in an HMO through his employer, but he had not seen a physician in several years. Metastatic prostate cancer, ureteral obstruction, and chronic renal failure were diagnosed. The patient's mental status improved, but he lacked decision-making capacity. His physicians recommended orchiectomy as palliative treatment, but two of Mr. Schmidt's family members disagreed with each other over the issue of the surgery. The ethics consultant was asked: "Should this incompetent patient receive an operation he needs but which is refused by a family member?"

The consultant spoke with the resident physicians and family members, including the patient's nephew who happened to be an attorney. Mr. Schmidt had not previously discussed treatment preferences, and had not previously refused any other medical treatment. The patient's brother, who had seen him almost weekly for many years, said he believed that the patient would want the surgery. The patient's nephew, however, asserted that the patient would not want the operation. He lived in, and stood to gain, the patient's house and had considered initiating legal procedures to declare the patient incompetent to manage his financial assets. Both the brother and the nephew stood to benefit from the patient's will.

Because of the family disagreement and suspicion regarding the nephew's motives, the consultant advised the patient's brother to obtain legal guardianship for health care and financial decisions. The court granted guardianship to the brother and prohibited the nephew from visiting the patient in the hospital. Mr. Schmidt was operated on and discharged to his brother's home to convalesce.

Here, the consultant addressed a financial conflict of interest that affected a proxy's judgment about the treatment of an incompetent patient. This role is a proper one for physicians, but is new. Physicians have tended to view socioeconomic considerations in patient care as external to ethical decision making.[38,83] This is perhaps because of a tradition of self-identification as their patients' primary advocate, fear of becoming agents of an inequitable distribution of social resources, or a sense of relatively unrestricted access to medical care through third-party payers.

In a recent study of 562 consecutive patient visits to a medical office, however, 56 ethical problems involving medical care costs were present.[84] Even though MCO cost constraints are widely discussed, our experience suggests that the economic motivation underlying requests for ethics consultation may not be apparent or may even be concealed in the consultation request. As the foregoing cases illustrate, financial constraints also may often arise from sources outside the MCO, such as the family or the community. Careful inquiry by the ethics consultant will often unmask the complex financial aspects of the dilemma. Once these economic aspects are uncovered, there are several ways in which ethics consultants can assist MCO physicians—and in which physicians can ethically take into account financial information—in ethical decision making.

Quality Assurance/Utilization Management: A Moral Necessity in Managed Care

As *quality* has become a buzzword in health care, major, scientifically based, process-oriented efforts at continuously improving quality have been initiated.[85] Quality of care research has evolved from an outcomes-oriented movement to one concerned with process and outcome, with a call for the implementation of practice guidelines and uniform standards for practice.[86,87]

Quality assurance committees attempt to ensure high-quality, appropriate care. MCOs assume that QA is a moral good and that increased scrutiny of doctor-patient outcomes can and will result in better medical care. The goals of QA are educationally driven and outcome-based: structure and process are important only if they improve patient outcome and change physician behavior.[75] Quality assurance focuses on providing "medically necessary" services; it is important to MCOs that QA does not become a euphemism for utilization management (UM).[88]

Many physicians already believe that the pursuit of quality is simply another money-saving method for MCOs, rather than a happy by-product of total quality improvement. *Quality* is a more attractive term than *utilization*: in 1990, after 20 years, the American College of Utilization Review Physicians changed its name to the American College of Medical Quality.

Mehlman notes four key criticisms of QA:

1. Defining quality care is difficult without adequate data.
2. Focusing on a few providers instead of overall care is ineffective, cumbersome, and biased.

3. Standardizing criteria for quality reviewers has not been sanctioned.
4. Paying for QA systems is burdensome.[89]

Stevens notes, "Defining quality in terms of norms extends decision making beyond traditional practitioners, and beyond their professional and hospital associations, to the realm of mechanistic management decisions."[90]

Despite interest in the deployment of managed care in state and federal health care reform packages, there are significant methodologic problems of measuring necessity and quality, determining patient satisfaction, and interpreting outcome data;[91,92] there are also ethical dilemmas of justice, autonomy, advocacy, fidelity, and confidentiality.

To circumvent quality assurance, and in place of appealing financial constraints on patient care, physicians may balance their patients' interests with MCO regulations by simply "gaming the system."[68] For example, doctors may note a "worrisome appearance" of a facial lesion so that a patient can see a dermatologist. They may annually "palpate" the breast lump of a 45-year-old woman, or fabricate a symptom in a preventive care checkup. They may also retrospectively "precertify" an emergency department visit for a patient who was too sick to call for permission first, or renew a hospital order to continue an intravenous line for an elderly patient in need of (but without MCO authorization for) further observation. While "massaging" the details of a case may help a patient gain access to care, it also diminishes professional credibility, and can lead other clinicians astray. Such a deception "can harm patients and society, offend honesty, and violate basic principles of contractual and distributive justice. It is also, in fact, usually unnecessary in securing needed resources for patients."[68]

Defining "medically necessary" care is important but difficult.[93,94] Approaches used by MCOs include patient satisfaction surveys, cost-effectiveness analyses, and legal experience.[95,96] An MCO patient with Gaucher's disease but without access to enzyme replacement replied to a *New York Times* essay on utilization management[97] by noting that the ultimate in cost-effectiveness for her MCO would be her death.[98] Another patient sued and won her case after she was prematurely discharged because UM suggested it.[27] Yet another patient's death prompted an appeals court to order a review company to stand trial, finding "this is a case where a cost-limitation program was permitted to corrupt medical judgment."[99]

Although UM is designed to promote quality care, physicians view it differently. The American Medical Association reports that 20 percent of over 4,000 physicians surveyed found UM to be the single factor that interferes most with clinical decision making; for internists, the figure was 30 percent. Preadmission or preprocedure certification and retrospective review were named as the most intrusive and most time consuming.[100] Practitioners also report disagreements among peer reviewers about what comprises appropriate care,[101] uncertainty about reviewer qualifications,[66] and uneasiness about reviewer requests for confidential patient information.[102] Doctors feel that UM forces them to choose between being a patient advocate and an MCO agent.[103]

Nevertheless, UM performs important functions: it attempts to assess the appropriateness of diagnostic and therapeutic modalities for individual MCO members and to ensure that members do not receive unnecessary services. UM can screen and exclude cost-outliers: MCO physician-gatekeepers who "overspend," thus posing a conflict of interest for these physicians,[104,105] who have financial incentives to restrict access and professional motivations to provide care. UM, however, is hampered by difficulties in defining and measuring quality, the uncertain relationship between quality and satisfaction, and lack of popular appeal.

New Ethical Responsibilities for Patients and Physicians in Managed Care

As illustrated in the foregoing cases and discussion, MCO patients and physicians have several new responsibilities. These are suggested by the cases, but it is important to list them explicitly as well:

1. As individuals, patients must take greater charge of their own health, especially to prevent diseases for which they are at special risk.
2. As MCO members, patients must acknowledge their decision to forgo some explicitly excluded services or to pay for them out-of-pocket. They must also acknowledge that the MCO will work to disallow expensive treatments, even if they are not explicitly excluded.
3. Patients, along with their doctors, must be responsible for appealing unfair economic constraints on their care, beginning with their point of MCO entry (often their place of employment).
4. As members of society, MCO members have civic responsibilities to speak in public health debates, including those on access to basic care.

Physicians also have several new responsibilities:

1. Physicians must be able to function as financial advocates while maintaining good professional relationships with their patients under managed care; if they cannot, managed care will ultimately fail.
2. Physicians must become more informed about their patients' MCO policies, so they can identify areas of interference and red tape, discern what is medically indicated from what is medically available, and use the gatekeeper role[106,107] to patient advantage.
3. Referrals to specialists, preauthorizations for surgery or hospitalization, and required follow-up visits all are within a gatekeeper's control.[108,109] Primary physicians should develop this role into one of clinical authority,[110] and take it on as a mantle of advocacy.[111,112]

Policymakers who create and offer managed care plans to the public must fully identify and disclose managed care's ethical assumptions. Reconciling individual variability and preferences with managed care's efforts at standardization will be difficult. Such standardized protocols, however, have immediate bedside implications for doctors and patients, as discussed previously.

MANAGED CARE AND MANAGED COMPETITION IN THE CLINTON ADMINISTRATION

Managed Care As the Future of the System

Most attempts at state and federal health care reform rely on managed care systems to deliver basic, standard medical care at a discounted, fixed price. Furthermore, managed care holds a prominent, critical place in the recent evolution of health policy, an evolution characterized in part by "bureaucratic parsimony"[113,114] or, more charitably, financial assessment and accountability.[115,116] Proposals for MCO enrollment of the Medicare[117] and Medicaid[118] populations have been given top priority by the Health Care Financing Administration (HCFA). Most proposals for overhauling the health care system feature managed care methods[119]— and reasonably so—for improved access, responsible cost containment, and effective quality assurance are central to national health care reform.[120-123] President Clinton's initial reform plans are to strengthen the MCO model and move toward "putting people first" with a managed competition approach.

Managed competition was defined by President Clinton in the *New England Journal of Medicine*[124] as combining

> an appropriate and revised governmental role with a reliance on the private sector to provide care and to compete to serve every person in this country. But that competition must take place under a restructured set of ground rules that foster competition to provide the best care at the best price, not to avoid covering the less healthy and to raise prices fastest for the sickest.

It includes an overall structure to contain costs and ensure access; a core benefit package; universal health benefits coverage; health networks, insurance reform; special provisions for small employers; medical malpractice reform; and slowed price increases on prescription drugs. Space does not permit an extensive review and analysis of managed competition's many details, but the reader will recognize that the heart of managed competition is managed care. The ethical assumptions of managed competition are the same as those in managed care.

President Clinton made a number of statements about managed competition on the campaign trail, and at the time of this writing he has not yet fully implemented any of his strategies. Some of the changes he proposes, however, will certainly occur and will have an impact on the future and the overall milieu of managed care. In the past, managed care was always an alternative to the overarching, dominant, highly capitalistic, fee-for-service system. Clinton demands that government make more of the rules, i.e., "manage" the competition. His initial plans are to reform the entire system along the lines of managed care.

He would establish a National Health Board made up of health care professionals and others to develop a core benefits package, as well as global budgets. Practice guidelines would be developed. Claims forms would be standardized. Drug prices would be cut. These practical features of cost containment have already been piloted and implemented in managed care. Overall budgets, core benefits, practice guidelines, standardized paperwork, and medication profiles are already part of managed care.

Furthermore, Clinton has endorsed the crucial concept of expenditure targets. Health care would be allowed to comprise only a certain percentage of the federal budget. This is managed care on a national level. While he is willing to allow variation in systems, he favors a play-or-else model that relies more heavily on managed care than any system to date. This model has been endorsed by both political parties, along with the Blues (Blue Cross and Blue Shield), hospital groups, business leaders, and major news publications.

Managed competition would combine consumers and providers into large HMO-like organizations. The government would use tax incentives to move people toward the system. It would also set the basic benefit package in the same manner as the administration of a mega-MCO. Provider plans would then have a quality-controlled price war for the business of large purchasing groups. The Clinton plan would require all employers to offer health insurance and pay at least some of the cost. Smaller employers would be able to buy through regional purchasing groups.[125]

Clinton would expand Medicare benefits to include phased-in long-term care, but again, under the restriction of global budgets and spending caps. He has not suggested any change in the Medicaid program. He would encourage care networks to coordinate care and reform antitrust statutes to increase provider cooperation. He advocates eliminating pre-existing conditions clauses from contracts, replacing experience rating with community rating, and increasing funding for AIDS research and prevention. His malpractice reform favors alternative dispute resolution mechanisms on a state-by-state basis.

Limitations of Managed Competition

A discussion of managed competition must acknowledge its several obvious limitations. A restructuring of the health care system will take many years to accomplish (probably into the 21st century), and may not control costs initially if other cost control measures are not vigorously initiated. For example, health care costs, if not controlled, will double in six years to more than 1.5 trillion dollars yearly. Another limitation is that a managed competition unit would require an estimated 200,000 to 500,000 health care consumers for a critical mass. In most rural areas, physicians and hospitals cannot generate the level of competition on which the model relies.[126] Finally, without careful attention to the ethical underpinnings of managed care, managed competition risks the same problems as a poorly run MCO. It risks being viewed as a high-paperwork, low-touch/low-care system concerned more with cost constraints than with equitable, quality medical care. It risks being seen as a system in which quality assurance is just another way to coerce patients and providers into compliance with low-level care. The ethical assumptions of managed care must be incorporated into managed competition.

CONCLUSION

The ethical and economic aspects of treatment decisions are intimately entwined.[127] Physicians can no longer ignore the effect of financial constraints on clinical decision making, as some ethicists have suggested they do.[128]

The goal of good medical practice is best served by acknowledging the influence of economic realities on clinical practice. Physicians should be aware of the ethical issues posed by financial constraints on patient care. Ethics consultation can at times be useful in the managed care setting.

Patients should be informed of conflicts of interest and the impact of these financial constraints on treatment recommendations and patient care. Professional advocacy means that physicians should assist patients with financial issues that are unreasonable, discriminatory, or detrimental to patients' medical interests.

Medicine's traditional ethic insists on patient and professional advocacy. By working with individual patients—a clinical effort—physicians can make systemic differences. By empowering patients and working with them to maintain the trust underlying the doctor-patient relationship, physicians can join with their most important allies. By acknowledging and studying their proliferating roles in the managed care system, physicians can better define and fulfill them.[101] By advocating disease prevention, health promotion, patient education, and a broad perspective on health care issues, physicians can encourage patient-minded QA and UM committees and MCO boards. By identifying the ethical assumptions of managed care, physicians, managers, and policymakers can better analyze and resolve them.

A simple cost containment agenda is neither physicians' nor patients' preferred course of action. The promises of managed care and managed competition depend on equal access, disease prevention, and health promotion, but the economic pressures of the current health care environment threaten to distort these concepts and destroy the fidelity of the doctor-patient relationship. If this happens, patients will suffer and managed care systems will collapse. This would be unfortunate, because equality of access, responsible cost-containment, and effective quality assurance are worthwhile goals for any health care organization. For MCOs, and the larger system of managed competition, achieving these goals will require honesty and fidelity—the same virtues embodied in the doctor-patient relationship.

REFERENCES

1. Mayer TR, Mayer GG. HMOs: origins and development. *N Engl J Med.* 1985;312:590–594.

2. Ellwood PM, Anderson NN, Billings JE, Carlson RJ, Hoagber EJ, McClure W. Health maintenance strategy. *Med Care.* 1971;9:291–298.

3. Hornbrook MC, Goodman MJ. Managed care: penalties, autonomy, risk and integration. In: Hibbard H, Nutting PA, Grady ML, eds. *Primary Care Research: Theory and Methods.* Washington,DC: U.S. Department of Health and Human Services; AHCPR 91–34, 1991:107–126.

4. Povar G, Moreno J. Hippocrates and the health maintenance organization: a discussion of the ethical issues. *Ann Intern Med.* 1988;109:419–424.

5. Himmelstein DU, Woolhandler S. The corporate compromise: a Marxist view of health maintenance organizations and prospective payment. *Ann Intern Med.* 1988; 109:494-501.

6. Wear S. Anticipatory ethical decision-making: the role of the primary physician. *HMO Practice.* 1989;3(2):41–46.

7. Hillman AL. Health maintenance organizations, financial incentives and physicians' judgments. *Ann Intern Med.* 1990;112:891–893.

8. Kane RA. Case management: ethical pitfalls on the road to high-quality managed care. *QRB.* May 1988:161–166.

9. Brook RH. Quality of care: do we care? *Ann Intern Med.* 1991;115:486–490.

10. Aaron HJ, Schwartz WB. *The Painful Prescription: Rationing Health Care.* Washington, DC: The Brookings Institution; 1984.

11. La Puma J, Lawlor E. Quality adjusted life years: implications for clinicians and policymakers. *JAMA.* 1990;263:2917–2921.

12. Mechanic D. The growth of HMOs: issues of enrollment and disenrollment. *Medical Care.* 1983;21:338–347.

13. Freidson E. The medical profession in transition. In: Aiken L, Mechanic D, eds. *Applications of Social Science to Clinical Medicine and Health Policy.* Trenton, NJ: Rutgers University Press; 1986.

14. Davies AR, Ware JE, Brook RH, Peterson JR, Newhouse JP. Consumer acceptance of prepaid and fee-for-service medical care: results from a randomized controlled trial. *Health Services Research.* 1986;3:429–452.

15. Welch WP, Miller M. Mandatory HMO enrollment in Medicaid: the issue of freedom of choice. *Milbank Q.* 1988;66:618–639.

16. Hillman AL. Financial incentives for physicians in HMOs: is there a conflict of interest? *N Engl J Med.* 1987;317:1743–1748.

17. Clancy DM, Hillner BE. Physicians as gatekeepers: the impact of financial incentives. *Arch Intern Med.* 1989;149:917–920.

18. Hillman AL, Pauly MV, Kerstein JJ. How do financial incentives affect physicians' clinical decisions and the financial performance of health maintenance organizations? *N Engl J Med.* 1989; 321:86–92.

19. Thurow LC. Medicine versus economics. *N Engl J Med.* 1985; 313:611–614.

20. Angell M. Cost containment and the physician. *JAMA.* 1985; 254:1203–1207.

21. Relman AS. Practicing medicine in the new business climate. *N Engl J Med.* 1987; 316:1150–1151.

22. Scovern H. A physician's experience in a for–profit staff model HMO. *N Engl J Med.* 1988;319:787–790.

23. *Wickline v. California*, 192 Cal. App. 3d 1630, 239 Cal. Rptr. 810 (1986).

24. *Sarchett v. Blue Shield of California*, 43 Cal.3d 1, 233 Cal. Rptr. 76, 729 P.2d 267 (1987).

25. Mayfield J, Grady ML, eds. *Conference Proceedings: Primary Care Research: An Agenda for the 90s.* Rockville, MD: The Agency for Health Services Research in Primary Care;1990: AHCPR 90–17.

26. Dorwart RA. Managed mental health care: myths and realities in the 1990s. *Hosp and Comm Psych.* 1990;41:1087–1091.

27. Welch WP, Hillman AL, Pauly MV. Toward new typologies for HMOs. *Milbank Q.* 1990;68(2):221–243.

28. Udvarhelyi IS, Jennison K, Phillips RS, Epstein AM. Comparison of the quality of ambulatory care for fee–for–service and prepaid patients. *Ann Intern Med.* 1991; 115:394–400.

29. Shulz R. Physician adaptation to health maintenance organizations and its implications for management. *Health Services Research.* 1990;25:43–63.

30. Morreim EH. Cost containment and the standard of medical care. *Calif Law Rev.* 1987;75:1719–1763.

31. Wennberg JE. Outcomes research: what does it really mean? *Managed Medicine.* 1991;2(1):7–13.

32. Goldfield N. Measurement and management of quality in managed care organizations: alive and improving. *QRB.* November 1991:343–348.

33. Brett AS. The case against persuasive advertising by health maintenance organizations. *N Engl J Med.* 1992;326:1353–1357.

34. Danis M, Churchill LR. Autonomy and the common weal. *Hastings Center Rept.* 1991; 21(1):25–31.

35. Belkin L. Doctors lose autonomy to health–care networks. *New York Times.* November 12, 1991;A1, B12.

36. Jonsen AR. *The New Medicine and the Old Ethics.* Cambridge, Mass: Harvard University Press; 1990.

37. Morreim EH. Cost containment: issues of moral conflict and justice for physicians. *Theor Med.* 1985;6:257–279.

38. Levinsky NG. The doctor's master. *N Engl J Med.* 1984;311:1573–1575.

39. Siegler M. The progression of medicine: from physicians paternalism to patient autonomy to bureaucratic parsimony. *Ann Intern Med.* 1985;145:713–715.

40. Kerns LL, Gerner C. A physician's guide to avoiding liability in managed care settings. *Chicago Medicine.* 1991;94(14):36–42.

41. La Puma J, Schiedermayer DL. Ethics consultation: skills, roles, and training. *Ann Internal Med.* 1992;114:155–160.

42. H.R. 939, 101st Cong., 1st Sess. (1989).

43. Morreim EH. Gaming the system: dodging the rules, ruling the dodgers. *Arch Internal Med.* 1991;151:443–447.

44. Levinson DF. Toward full disclosure of referral restrictions and financial incentives by prepaid health plans. *N Engl J Med.* 1987;317:1729–1731.

45. Ansell DA, Schiff RL. Patient dumping: status, implications, and policy recommendations. *JAMA.* 1987;257:1500–1502.

46. Schiff RL, Ansell DA, Schlosser JE, et al. Transfers to a public hospital: a prospective study of 467 patients. *N Engl J Med.* 1986;314:552–557.

47. La Puma J, Balskus M. When an indigent patient needs a helicopter: a case report and an accepted institutional policy. *J Emerg Med.* 1988;6:147–149.

48. Kellermann AL, Ackerman TF. Interhospital patient transfer: the case for informed consent. *N Engl J Med.* 1988;319:643–647.

49. Gray BH, Field MJ, eds. *Controlling costs and changing patient care? The role of utilization management.* Institute of Medicine Committee on Utilization Management by Third Parties. Washington, DC: National Academy Press;1989:1539.

50. Schneller ES. The leadership and executive potential of physicians in an era of managed care systems. *Hosp and Health Serv Admin.* 1991;36(1):43–55.

51. Schiedermayer DL, La Puma J, Miles SH. Ethics consultation masking economic dilemmas in patient care. *Arch Intern Med.* 1989; 149:1303–1305.

52. La Puma J, Cassel CK, Humphrey H. Ethics, economics and endocarditis: the physician's role in resource allocation. *Arch Intern Med.* 1988; 148;1809–1811.

53. Miles SH. Requested non beneficial treatment: the case of Helga Wanglie. *N Engl J Med.* 1991;325.

54. Redelmeier DA, Tversky A. Discrepancy between medical decisions for individual patients and for groups. *N Engl J Med.* 1990;322:1162–1164.

55. Levinson DF. Toward full disclosure of referral restrictions and financial incentives by prepaid health plans. *N Engl J Med.* 1987;317:1729–1731.

56. Ware JE Jr, Brook RH, Rogers WH, et al. Comparison of health outcomes at a health maintenance organization with those of fee–for–service care. *Lancet.* 1986;1:1017–1022.

57. Eddy DM. The challenge. *JAMA.* 1990;263:287–290.

58. Epstein AM, Begg CB, McNeil BJ. The use of ambulatory testing in prepaid and fee–for–service group practice: relations to perceived profitability. *N Engl J Med.* 1986;314:1089–1094.

59. Lundberg GD. How should physicians be paid? *JAMA.* 1985;254:2638–2639.

60. Ginzberg E. What lies ahead for American physicians: one economist's views. *JAMA.* 1985;253:2878–2879.

61. Relman AS, Reinhardt U. An exchange on for–profit health care. In: Gray BH, ed: *For–Profit Enterprise in Health Care.* Washington DC: Institute of Medicine. The National Academy Press; 1986.

62. Hillman AL. Financial incentives for physicians in HMOs: is there a conflict of interest? *N Engl J Med.* 1987;317:1743–1748.

63. Levinson DF. Toward full disclosure of referral restrictions and financial incentives by prepaid health plans. *N Engl J Med.* 1987;317:1729–1731.

64. Povar G, Moreno J. Hippocrates and the health maintenance organization. *Ann Intern Med.* 1988;109:419–424.

65. Blendon RJ, Donelan K. The emerging debate over national health insurance. *N Engl J Med.* 1990;323:208–212.

66. Bone RC. Honoring patient preferences and rationing intensive care: are these compatible goals? *Arch Intern Med.* 1991;151:1061–1063.

67. *Wickline v. California,* Second Appellate District, Div 5, July 30, 1986.

68. Wilensky GR, Rossiter LF. Patient self-selection in HMOs. *Health Affairs.* 1986; 5:66–80.

69. Pellegrino ED. Toward a reconstruction of medical morality: the primacy of profession and the fact of illness. *J Med Philos.* 1979;4:32–56.

70. Parsons T. *The Social System.* New York: Free Press; 1951.

71. Cassell EJ. The nature of suffering and the goals of medicine. *N Engl J Med.* 1982;306:639–645.

72. Stout CE. Managed care and the human touch: are they compatible? *Chicago Med.* 1992;95(18):24–27.

73. Ad Hoc Committee on Medical Ethics. American College of Physicians' Ethics Manual. *Ann Intern Med.* 1989;111: 242–252, 327–335.

74. Kass LR. *Toward a More Natural Science: Biology and Human Affairs.* New York: Free Press;1968:148.

75. Ende J, Kazis L, Ash A, Moskowitz MA. Measuring patients' desire for autonomy: decision-making and information-seeking preferences among medical patients. *J Gen Intern Med.* 1989;4:23–30.

76. Roter EL, Hall JA, Katz NR. Patient–physician communication: a descriptive summary of the literature. *Patient Education and Counseling.* 1988;1299–1319.

77. Quill TE. Recognizing and adjusting to barriers in doctor–patient communication. *Stern Med.* 1989;111:51–58.

78. Freundenheim M. Guarding medical confidentiality. *The New York Times.* January 1, 1991;24.

79. Borenstein DJ. Managed care: a means of rationing psychiatric treatment. *Hosp and Comm Psych.* 1990;41:1095–1098.

80. Siegler M. The physician-patient accommodation: a central event in clinical medicine. *Arch Intern Med.* 1982;142:1899–1902.

81. May WF. *The Physician's Covenant.* Philadelphia, Pa: The Westminster Press; 1983.

82. Kolata G. Wariness is replacing trust between healer and patient. *The New York Times.* ;October 20, 1990;A1, D15.

83. Siegler M. Decision-making strategy for clinical ethical problems in medicine. *Arch Intern Med.* 1982;142:2178–2179.

84. Connelly JE, Campbell C. Patients who refuse treatment in medical offices. *Arch Intern Med.* 1987;147:1829–1833.

85. Kritchevsky SB, Simmons BP. Continuous quality improvement: concepts and applications for physician care. *JAMA.* 1991;266:1817–1823.

86. Brook RH. Practice guidelines and practicing medicine: are they compatible? *JAMA.* 1989;262:3027–3030.

87. Woolf SH. Practice guidelines, a new reality in medicine: methods of developing guidelines. *Arch Intern Med.* 1991;152:946–952.

88. Adelman SH. Is quality assurance a euphemism for saving the payers money? *Am Med News.* October 5, 1990:18.

89. Mehlman MJ. Assuring the quality of medical care: the impact of outcome measurement and practice standards. *Law Med Health Care.* 1990;18(4):368–384.

90. Stevens R. *In sickness and in wealth: American hospitals in the twentieth century.* New York: Basic Books;1989:329.

91. Shortell SM, Hughes EFX. The effects of regulation, competition, and ownership on mortality rates among hospital inpatients. *N Engl J Med.* 1988;318:1100–1107.

92. Williams S. The limit of quantitative ethics. *Med Decis Making.* 1987;7:121–123.

93. Brook RH. Health, health insurance, and the uninsured. *JAMA.* 1991;265:2998–3002.

94. Aukerman GF. Access to health care for the uninsured: the perspective of the American Academy of Family Physicians. *JAMA.* 1991;265:2856–2858.

95. Emery DD, Schneiderman LJ. Cost-effectiveness analysis in health care. *Hastings Center Rept.* 1989;19(4):8–13.

96. Eisenberg JM. Clinical economics–a guide to the economic analysis of clinical practices. *JAMA.* 1989;262:2879–2886.

97. Kramon G. Medical second-guessing—in advance. *The New York Times.* February 24, 1991.

98. Shafarman L. The bane of medical second-guessing. *The New York Times.* March 3, 1991;3:9.

99. Freudenheim M. Doctors press states to curb review of procedures' costs. *The New York Times.* 1991;A1, C3.

100. Larkin H. Liability fears interfering with clinical decisions, physicians say. *Amer Med News.* April 22/29, 1991:11.

101. Grumbach K, Bodenheimer T. Reins or fences: a physician's view of cost containment. *Health Affairs.* Winter 1990:120–126.

102. Goyal A. Utilization reviews: a strength carried to excess becomes a weakness. *Chicago Med.* 1991;94(9):4–5.

103. Abrams FR. Patient advocate or secret agent. *JAMA.* 1986;256:1784–1785.

104. Morreim EH. Conflicts of interest: profits and problems in physician referrals. *JAMA.* 1989;262:390–394.

105. Rodwin MA. Physicians conflicts of interest. *N Engl J Med.* 1990;321:1405–1408.

106. Reagan MD. Physicians as gatekeepers: a complex challenge. *N Engl J Med.* 1987;317:1731–1734.

107. Schiedermayer DL. The general internist as gatekeeper. *Ann Intern Med.* 1985;103:160.

108. Eisenberg J. The internist as gatekeeper. *Ann Intern Med.* 1985;102:537–543.

109. Berman HS, Rose L. *Choosing the Right Health Care Plan.* Mt. Vernon, New York: Consumers Union; 1990:170–171.

110. Cassel CK. The general internist and gatekeepers. *Ann Intern Med.* 1985;103:160.

111. Kleinman LC. Health care in crisis: a proposed role for the individual physician as an advocate. *JAMA.* 1991;265:1991–1992.

112. Moore C. Need for a patient advocate. *JAMA.* 1989;262:259–260.

113. Siegler M. The progression of medicine: from physician paternalism to patient autonomy to bureaucratic parsimony. *Arch Intern Med.* 1985;145:713–715.

114. Sack K. Albany budget plan calls for managed care to cut Medicaid costs. *The New York Times.* May 31, 1991;A14.

115. Relman AS. Assessment and accountability. *N Engl J Med.* 1988;319:1220–1222.

116. Detsky AS, Naglie IG. A clinician's guide to cost–effectiveness analysis. *Ann Intern Med.* 1990;113:147–154.

117. Iglehart JK. Medicare turns to HMOs. *N Engl J Med.* 1986;312:123–126.

118. Burke M. State managed care initiatives spur Medicaid policy debate. *Hospitals.* August 20, 1991;46–52.

119. *JAMA.* 1991;265:1213–1340.

120. Nutter DO, Helms CM, Whitcomb ME, Weston WD. Restructuring health care in the United States: a proposal for the 1990s. *JAMA.* 1991;265:2516–2520.

121. Rockefeller JD IV. A call for action: the Pepper Commission's blueprint for health care reform. *JAMA.* 1991;265:2507–2510.

122. Health and Public Policy Committee, American College of Physicians. Access to health care. *Ann Intern Med.* 1990;112:641–662.

123. The Right Medicine. Op–Ed. *The New York Times.* May 27, 1991;A1:16.

124. Clinton B. The Clinton health care plan. *N Engl J Med*. 1992;327:804–807.

125. *American Medical News*. November 23,30, 1992:1, 46.

126. Simmons HE, Rhoades MM, Goldberg MA. Comprehensive health care reform and managed competition. *N Engl J Med*. 1992;327(21):1525–1527.

127. Agich GJ. Incentives and obligations under prospective payment. *J Med Phil*. 1987;12:123–144.

128. Veatch RM. *A Theory of Medical Ethics*. New York: Basic Books; 1981:285.

Editorial Commentary

Susan L. Howell

David B. Nash

Many managed care physicians feel torn between the economic considerations of the practice versus the well-being of the patient. This scenario exemplifies one of the most popular arguments against managed care. That we should have difficulty adjusting to the "logic" of managed care—enhanced quality at reduced costs—and struggle with concomitant ethical dilemmas is understandable, given the tenets of traditional practice.

Authors John La Puma and David Schiedermayer, both physician ethicists, one at a community teaching hospital and one at the Medical College of Wisconsin, explore in detail the ethics of managed care. Through their careful analysis and attention to the hard questions prompted by managed care, we begin to more thoroughly understand its ethical foundation, and how an awareness of this ethical foundation can help physicians maintain consistently high standards for compassionate care.

Drs. La Puma and Schiedermayer represent the next generation of physician ethicists who evaluate many of the issues surrounding current "perverse" incentives within both the prepaid and fee-for-service sectors. Ethical considerations inevitably arise as a result of the incentive systems in managed care, and exist at both the interphysician level (issues of professional sovereignty, conflicts of interest) as well as the doctor-patient level. In this chapter, the authors go beyond the ethical ramifications of well-described financial incentives to those regarding access to care, specific technologies, and rationing of services.

Drs. La Puma and Schiedermayer begin with a review of the pros and cons of managed care from the perspectives of patients, physicians, and insurers, and identify the ethical assumptions underlying good managed care. They present case studies to illustrate some typical ethical dilemmas encountered in the managed care setting and discuss the role of the ethics consultant in mediating a solution. The authors also have undertaken the task of prophesizing about our imminent health care future under the

Clinton administration, focusing on Clinton's proposed managed competition model. In this ethical and practical context, we are presented with a "snapshot" of what we, as managed health care professionals, can expect our newly assumed roles and responsibilities to be.

The authors warn against overzealous attention to economic considerations in the absence of contemplative evaluation of all facets and potential outcomes of the patient encounter. This requires an openness to acquiring new skills and learning new ways of thinking for which traditional training historically has not prepared us. Attention to managed care's "moral mission" is essential if we are to successfully navigate the challenges that lie ahead. It is also our best insurance, as individuals, for carrying out our daily duties with efficiency and peace of mind.

Chapter 4

Leadership in Managed Care Organizations: The Role of the Physician Manager

Harry L. Leider
Marc A. Bard

A VISIT TO THE QUALITY HEALTHCARE PLAN

"Quality Healthcare Plan" is a large staff-model health maintenance organization in Metropolis, USA. Hundreds of physicians, nurses, and assistants provide medical care to over 300,000 patients in 10 new and inviting health centers. Quality Healthcare is a dynamic and growing HMO managed by a partnership of physicians and professional managers who work together to help the Plan deliver its missions of "excellent care at a reasonable cost." Let's take a brief look at some of the issues and challenges faced by a few of Quality Healthcare's physician managers in a typical week.

Doctor Sarah Smith—Chief of Internal Medicine

At the Downtown Health Center, the Chief of Internal Medicine, Sarah Smith, MD, leads a weekly meeting of the doctors and nurses in her department. The major topic of the day is Dr. Smith's desire to set some clinical goals for her department for the coming year. During the hour meeting, she asks the group to brainstorm ideas for clinical goals. She then helps the group generate a list of over 30 ideas ranging from improving influenza immunization rates to reducing cholesterol levels in patients at high risk for coronary artery disease.

Dr. Smith facilitates a group discussion of the relative merits of the various suggestions. She then conducts a vote and the group selects three goals: to increase the number of women who receive routine mammograms, to increase the number of patients who quit smoking, and to improve the control of blood pressure in hypertensive patients. Finally, Dr. Smith appoints three committees to study these issues and to make recommendations to the department about how to achieve these goals.

Dr. John Jones—Medical Director

Later that week, the medical director of Downtown Health Center, Dr. John Jones, meets with Dr. Smith to discuss the rapid rise in hospital costs for patients enrolled at their health center. Dr. Jones asks Dr. Smith if there are any ways to care for some hospitalized patients in an outpatient setting. Together they review a list of the most frequent diagnoses for patients admitted to the medical service. Dr. Smith notes that the data show that a frequent reason for admission to the hospital is severe exacerbation of asthma. She acknowledges that recent advances in asthma treatment, such as more aggressive use of inhaled corticosteroids and enhanced patient education, have not filtered down to all the clinicians in her department. She believes that these new strategies have the potential to decrease hospitalizations.

Dr. Barry Barnes—Director of Clinical Guidelines

Dr. Jones informs Dr. Smith that a group of physicians in Quality Healthcare's department of clinical guidelines is developing a new guideline for the treatment of chronic asthma. He suggests that Dr. Smith contact Dr. Barry Barnes, the director of the clinical guidelines department, to see if this guideline could assist the clinicians in her department adopt new practices to help asthma patients avoid hospitalization. Dr. Smith returns to her office and after an enjoyable and busy afternoon of seeing patients, she calls Dr. Barnes.

Dr. Barnes enthusiastically relates that his department recently completed a new guideline on asthma. It does in fact highlight recent advances in the treatment of asthma. He offers to integrate this guideline into a one-hour CME program for the clinicians in Dr. Smith's department. Dr. Smith agrees that this would be a good approach. Dr. Barnes will develop the program and one of the physicians who developed the guideline will present it to Dr. Smith's department in two months.

Dr. Cathy Chen—Staff Pediatrician

The next day, Dr. Cathy Chen finishes a challenging morning of pediatric practice at the downtown center. She enjoyed seeing a thrilled mother bring her newborn girl to her office for the first checkup. She also saw a five-year-old child who was not gaining weight as expected. Dr. Chen spent a great deal of time evaluating this young patient and reassuring the worried parents that the child was healthy but required a change in diet. After Dr. Chen finishes her morning practice session she joins the rest of her practice team for a lunchtime team meeting.

As their elected team leader, Dr. Chen is responsible for helping the team's four physicians, two nurses, and three medical assistants work together efficiently and effectively to provide care to the team's patients. The topic for today's meeting is to plan the team's clinical schedules for the upcoming winter holiday season. Before the meeting, Dr. Chen wrote some key questions on the conference room's blackboard: How many doctors and nurses do we need in the office over the holidays? Do we need more clinicians in the office on the traditionally busy day after a holiday weekend? If we don't have enough "volunteers" to cover the practice, how will we decide who will work?

In the early part of the meeting, Dr. Chen leads the team through a discussion of these questions. The answers become the principles they use later in the meeting to negotiate with each other about vacation plans. Dr. Chen then facilitates the team negotiations and helps the group create a schedule. The result is a schedule that all team members feel is fair and ensures that the office is adequately staffed during the holiday season.

This fictional account quickly illustrates a few of the interesting and important management roles for physicians in today's managed care organizations. In this chapter we attempt to answer the following questions:

1. Why do some physicians choose to incorporate management or leadership responsibilities into their career?
2. Why do managed care organizations need good physician managers?
3. What types of management or leadership roles can physicians assume?

4. What are the critical management skills or competencies that physicians need to acquire to be effective in their new roles as managers?
5. How can physicians acquire and develop these competencies and start to use them in managerial and leadership roles?

In addition, we attempt to forecast the future role of physician managers in managed care organizations as our health care system evolves over the next five to ten years.

WHY PHYSICIANS BECOME MANAGERS

Until about 10 or 15 years ago, if you asked the average physician why any doctor would choose to go into management, the traditional response was that a physician went into management only for a more relaxed life-style or to flee the rigors of clinical medicine. Management roles were primarily titular or liaison positions that lacked real authority or responsibility. These positions were a steppingstone to retirement, or a safe haven for doctors who failed to build successful practices. It was inconceivable that a bright, successful clinician would choose to move into management and limit or eliminate his or her clinical practice.

The American College of Physician Executives (ACPE)

This conventional view of physician managers is clearly antiquated and erroneous. A national survey of physician managers in many different organizations (e.g., hospitals, HMOs, group practices, etc.) conducted in 1986 by the ACPE, a professional organization of physician managers, found that the most common reasons that physicians moved into management were a desire to be challenged, to lead others, to achieve more professional growth, and to maintain continued autonomy.[1] In addition, the majority of respondents saw participation in management as a way to have an impact on many people and to participate in important health policy decisions. Financial rewards were felt to be unimportant incentives for most of the physicians surveyed.

The survey also asked the same physician managers what their major goals were when they made the transition from practice to management. Although their responses varied considerably, common themes included the desire to improve health care services and to be part of the changes occurring in our health care system. Many physicians also expressed the desire to achieve new opportunities for personal and professional growth and satisfaction. Also of interest is that physicians seemed satisfied with their decision to become managers; 80 percent planned to remain in management and 96 percent were somewhat or very satisfied with their management roles.

Although this survey was not limited to physicians in managed care organizations, it is our impression that physicians in managed care organizations seek management and leadership opportunities for reasons similar to those cited in the survey. To confirm our impressions, we conducted a series of informal interviews with a group of physician managers in selected managed care organizations throughout the country. Their reasons for entering management were remarkably consistent with the results of the survey conducted by the ACPE.

Desire To Improve Health Care

The desire to improve health care services was a consistent theme. One chief of medicine said, "I saw so many problems that needed to be solved that I decided to get involved and make management part of my career." A director of a large health center remarked, "I had a need to plan and fix things. I initially served as a team leader and I enjoyed the opportunity to identify problems and improve the environment of my team."

Desire To Influence Others

Another consistent response was the desire to influence a larger number of people. A medical director of a group model HMO said, "I became energized by what management could provide to others and to me. I wanted to have a greater impact on more people." A health center director in a staff-model HMO said, "I wanted to have increased control and impact." Another medical director related, "I had ideas I wanted to see implemented and management just crept up on me. "

Desire To Develop Policy

A final common thread in our conversations was the desire to be involved in larger health policy issues. Most of the physician managers we talked with wanted to participate in improving our health care system and saw management as a way to achieve this goal. For example, a regional medical director in a mixed model HMO said, "I think it's important for physicians to become involved in the larger policy issues in health care." He saw his leadership role in a managed care organization as a way of participating in problem solving within the health care system.

Interestingly, none of these individuals saw management as a way to avoid clinical practice. Most commented that they viewed their participation in management as a way to enrich their careers and professional lives. Despite the slightly higher salaries of physician managers versus full-time primary care clinicians, only one of our respondents mentioned money as a motivating factor for pursuing a management career.

MANAGED CARE ORGANIZATIONS NEED GOOD PHYSICIAN MANAGERS

A useful definition of managed care is "an approach that superimposes structure, control, measurement, and accountability upon the health care system to effect a balance in the utilization of health care resources, cost containment, and quality enhancement."[2] Managed care has become a major force in our health care system and many health economists are promoting "competitive managed care" as a unifying model for the future of American health care.[3]

One of the results of the rapid growth of managed care is the interest and enthusiasm regarding the new role of the physician manager or physician executive.[4-9] Hospitals, group practices, ambulatory clinics, industrial corporations, insurance companies, and the government are turning to physician managers to help these organizations succeed in the increasingly competitive health care marketplace.

Nowhere is the role of physician manager more vital and dynamic than within managed care organizations. To see why this is true, several key factors must be considered: the central role of physicians in determining the cost and quality of health care; the traditional orientation and training of physicians; the mission of the managed care organization; and finally, the "clash of cultures"[10] between the traditional role of physicians and the goals and functioning of today's managed care organizations.

The Central Role of Physicians—Cost and Quality

Although many factors influence the cost and quality of health care delivered by an organization, the dominant force is the clinical decisions made by physicians. For example, the single decision of whether to admit a patient with atypical chest pain to the hospital to "rule out" a myocardial infarction can have a dramatic positive impact on the patient's health if the patient is having a heart attack. On the other hand, this decision can commit thousand of dollars to evaluating a patient with simple heartburn. Similarly, the decisions of whether to order a magnetic resonance imaging scan for a patient with a severe headache and a normal neurologic exam, or whether to treat a patient with AIDS with an expensive experimental antiviral drug have parallel implications regarding the trade-off between the patient's health and the cost of care.

Physicians make countless decisions like these every day. Not every one is as critical to a patient's health or as costly as the two examples stated above. Nonetheless, each decision or action contributes to the cost and quality of medical care. One school of thought supports the notion that physicians should not worry about costs because their fiduciary role is to seek improved health status for their patients. Following this paradigm to an extreme would suggest that physicians should admit *any* patient with chest pain to the hospital because there is always a small, but real chance that the patient has a life-threatening illness. Obviously, this does not happen. It is clear that to some degree, physicians have always confronted trade-offs between cost and quality. Nonetheless, physicians historically paid minimal attention to the costs of health care services.

The Traditional Training and Orientation of Physicians

We believe that the training and orientation of physicians emphasizes developing "a fund of clinical knowledge" and technical skills, seeking improved health status for individual patients regardless of cost, maintaining professional autonomy, and practicing alone. During medical school and residency training, physicians learn to admire the prodigious fund of clinical knowledge of their attending physicians. Similarly, in tertiary hospitals they are exposed to a dazzling array of medical technologies and interventions. The young physician quickly learns to believe that "quality" in medical care consists of using the most advanced diagnostic and therapeutic modalities in almost every situation.

Until recently, the dominant mode of financing health care was fee-for-service. Within a fee-for-service environment physicians have financial incentives to provide more services (e.g., hospital admissions, tests, medications, etc.) to a patient even when the chance of improving the patient's health status is small or unknown. Also, the use (and probable overuse) of expensive medical procedures and treatments by physicians is reinforced.

Physicians have traditionally viewed autonomy as an important and desirable characteristic of medical practice. The medical profession holds a special and revered place in our society and until recently, physicians have retained a high level of autonomy and control over their professional lives. In fact, it is our impression that many physicians view the autonomy of the profession as an important factor in their decision to pursue a career in medicine.

Finally, physicians generally work alone. Even physicians who work in large multispecialty groups frequently practice medicine in relative isolation. They may refer patients to their colleagues or to allied health professionals on a regular basis. Nonetheless, they rarely collaborate to develop better and more cost-effective strategies to care for patients.

The Mission of Managed Care Organizations

In contrast, as stated earlier, managed care seeks to achieve a balance between controlling health care costs and potentially enhancing quality of care. A more positive way of stating this is that managed care seeks to achieve the highest quality of care at the lowest cost. To achieve this mission, physicians within managed care organizations must make clinical decisions taking into account both the potential health benefits to the patient and the potential cost to the organization (and, ultimately, to patients enrolled in the managed care plan).

The "Clash of Cultures"

Physicians are not well prepared to accept this responsibility. In fact there is a fundamental "clash of cultures" between the goals and functioning of managed care organizations and the traditional orientation and training of physicians.[10] It is the need to manage this dynamic tension that provides the physician manager with a unique set of opportunities, challenges, and rewards in managed care organizations.

For example, although acquiring and maintaining technical skills is important for managed care physicians, it is important to the organization that physicians use these skills appropriately. Recent studies suggest that approximately one-quarter to two-thirds of many common medical interventions (e.g., upper gastrointestinal [GI] endoscopy, carotid endarterectomy, coronary angiography, coronary bypass surgery, etc.) are unnecessary or inappropriate.[11-13] To effectively manage care, HMOs require physicians to provide expensive services and use their technical skills only when there is a reasonable chance that patients will substantially benefit from the interventions.

A similar conflict exists regarding professional autonomy. Managed care organizations require that physicians work within a structured system. Physicians usually refer patients to specific hospitals, specialists, and laboratories. Use of expensive tests, medications, or procedures may require special approval from specialists within the organization.

In addition to asking physicians to work within a structured system, managed care organizations challenge the autonomy of physicians by trying to decrease variation in their practice styles.

For example, when evaluating an adult patient with dyspepsia, physicians have a significant number of diagnostic and therapeutic options. Physicians can choose to order an upper GI X-ray series, obtain an upper GI endoscopy, empirically treat with antacids, or empirically treat with H–2 antagonists. Clinicians can defend each of these options as good medical practice and each has different implications with respect to cost. It is also not clear whether the more aggressive (and expensive) diagnostic approaches actually improve health outcomes.

When facing an array of options like those mentioned above, physicians demonstrate great variation in their decisions and practice styles. With the goal of optimizing the relationship between quality and cost, managed care organizations attempt to decrease this variation by having physicians commit to practicing in a uniform way for a given medical condition. Managed care organizations have tried two generic approaches to accomplish this: clinical rules and incentives.[14]

Clinical Rules and Incentives

There are several types of clinical rules. Practice guidelines, clinical algorithms, utilization reviews, and administrative restrictions are only a few of the common strategies organizations use to communicate rules to its health care providers. Clinical rules are often constructed by a panel of clinical "experts" who work within the managed care organization. Alternatively, many national organizations create clinical rules that are available to managed care organizations. An example of a clinical rule (in this case a "guideline") for the example of dyspepsia is that young adults with new onset dyspepsia without complications of bleeding, weight loss, or dysphagia should be treated empirically with H–2 antagonists and should not receive an X-ray or upper endoscopy unless they fail medical therapy.

Another more flexible strategy for decreasing variation in practice is the use of incentives. Incentives are usually financial and reward physicians for practicing in a cost-effective manner. Health care organizations can construct incentives in a number of ways. Capitation payments, bonus distributions, and withhold accounts for specialty services are a few of the more common incentive systems used in managed care.

Let's return to our example of the variation in practice styles for evaluating and treating patients with dyspepsia. Some managed care plans provide physicians with an incentive to order fewer expensive procedures, such as endoscopy, by providing a bonus at the end of the year based on the financial performance of the plan. Other organizations withhold a portion of the physician's compensation during the year and return a variable amount of the money to the physician based on his or her utilization of expensive specialty and diagnostic services.

There are advantages and disadvantages to both clinical rules and financial incentives. Clinical rules are often viewed by physicians as "cookbook medicine." They delineate precisely how a physician should act in a given clinical situation and therefore more directly challenge the autonomy of physicians to make clinical decisions. On the other hand, clinical rules provide guidance to physicians on how to act under conditions of uncertainty. This can lead to improved quality of care—in addition to lower costs.

Incentives provide physicians with much greater freedom to make decisions in specific clinical situations. Nonetheless, they do little to directly improve quality of care. In addition, they can create a conflict between physicians' fiduciary obligation to act on their patients' behalf and their responsibility to improve the financial position of the managed care organization. One expert suggests that by using a combination of rules and incentives, managed care organizations can simultaneously lower costs while improving quality of care.[14]

Managed care organizations also require that physicians and other health care providers work together to provide patients with high quality and cost-effective care. For example, an internist working in a traditional multispecialty group may refer a newly diagnosed diabetic patient with an infected toe to an emergency room. The patient is admitted to the hospital for intravenous antibiotics. After discharge the internist sends the patient to an endocrinologist to receive more instruction on maintaining adequate glucose control and to a podiatrist to receive instruction on foot care.

In an efficient managed care plan, the internist evaluates the patient in the office and arranges for a physician's assistant to start an intravenous line to administer antibiotics. An office supervisor arranges home intravenous antibiotic therapy, the internist starts the patient on insulin, and then refers the patient to a diabetes class to learn about diabetes and the specifics of diet, insulin use, and the importance of proper foot care. Finally, the internist, if unavailable the next day, might arrange for a colleague to reevaluate the patient in the office the next day.

The traditional orientation and training of physicians and the goals and functioning of managed care organizations are frequently in conflict. Managing and resolving this "clash of cultures" is a unique opportunity and challenge for the physician manager in managed care. The physician's need for autonomy must be reconciled with the organization's need for structure, control, and accountability. The physician's need to use his or her skills to improve patients' health must be reconciled with the organization's need to use expensive services only when they are of proven added value. Lastly, physicians must alter their orientation to practice autonomously so that they can be part of an efficient and effective team that collaboratively delivers care to patients.

Physician managers are singularly qualified to manage these critical tensions. Their medical training allows them instinctual understanding of the needs and priorities of practicing physicians. Their management abilities allow them simultaneous understanding and acceptance of the organization's imperative of balancing individual patient needs with the broader needs of the plan's membership (e.g., reasonable premiums). Furthermore, the physician manager can communicate with both clinicians and nonclinical managers and help these two groups work together to achieve the mission of the organization.

To be successful, then, physician managers must effectively span the two cultures and reconcile the conflicts. They do this by empowering physicians and other health care professionals to maintain control over their professional lives despite the need for accountability and structure. Physician managers do this in several ways. They encourage clinicians and their staff to innovate and create new methods of organizing their clinical practices. These methods further the mission of their organizations while simultaneously meeting their individual needs. They work collaboratively with physicians and managers to build efficient systems that support the delivery of high quality and cost-effective care. Finally, they foster teamwork among health care providers, staff, and nonclinical managers.

Successful physician managers ultimately move beyond simply managing the conflicts. They recognize that the dynamic tensions between physicians and managed care organizations can be a positive force. These tensions, in part, provide the energy for managed care organizations' evolution. Successful physician managers embrace these conflicts and use them to challenge the organization and physicians to innovate and grow together. In this way, physician managers play a critical role in the evolution and development of managed care organizations.

WHAT MANAGEMENT AND LEADERSHIP ROLES ARE AVAILABLE TO PHYSICIANS IN MANAGED CARE ORGANIZATIONS?

The story about our fictional HMO illustrates the many different types of management and leadership roles available to physicians. The specific titles may vary from organization to organization but the responsibilities inherent in these positions remain relatively constant across different managed care plans. These roles represent various points along two dimensions—the *type* of management position and the *span of influence* of the position. The type of position describes the content of the physician's managerial role while the span of influence describes the breadth of management responsibility.

Type of Position

The type of position consists of four basic categories. *Line managers* directly or indirectly manage the staff and professionals who deliver medical care. Team leaders, chiefs of departments, and medical directors are examples of line manager positions. *Program managers* direct ongoing functions that support the delivery of health care. Programs that physicians commonly manage are departments of quality assurance or quality improvement, physician recruitment, CME, and teaching programs.

In addition to these traditional roles, managed care organizations are creating many new and innovative program leadership roles for physician managers. A few of these new roles include:

- creating and managing clinical databases
- directing risk management activities
- leading utilization management efforts
- organizing efforts to develop clinical rules

Project managers lead a time-limited project or committee directed at improving the quality or lowering the cost of medical care provided by the health care plan. Leading a task force to improve departmental methods of counseling patients who want to quit smoking, or directing an effort to reduce utilization of high cost pharmaceuticals are examples of project management roles. *Governing managers* participate within or lead a group that represents the professional interests of the physicians in the managed care plan. Serving as president of the physicians' organization or representing the physician group on the board of directors are examples of the governing roles physicians can assume.

Span of Influence

The span of influence refers to the size of the activity or group being managed. Span of influence means managing at the level of the team, department or specialty, health center, geographical region, or entire health care plan. Span of influence can vary considerably within these categories. For example, the chief of internal medicine in a large health center leading a group of 25 internists has a much larger span of influence than the center's chief of surgery who leads a group of four surgeons. The afore-mentioned categories help us to conceptualize the size of a physician's managerial responsibilities. Tables 4–1 and 4–2 list examples of the kind of positions available to physicians along the two dimensions of management and leadership.

Table 4–1 The Span of Influence in Line and Program Management

Span of Influence	Line Management	Program Management
Clinical Team	Internal Medicine Team Leader	Team Diabetes Education Coordinator Team Peer Review Coordinator Team Coordinator for Immunizations
Clinical Department	Chief of Pediatrics Associate Chief of Mental Health	Internal Medicine CME Coordinator Pediatric Coordinator for Student Programs Mental Health Peer Review Chairperson
Medical Center	Health Center Director Physician-in-Chief	Director of Emergency Response Team Director of Infection Control
Geographic Region	Regional Medical Director Regional Chief of Surgery	Regional Urgent Care Director Regional Home Care Coordinator
Health Care Plan	Medical Director President Chief Executive Officer	Director of Physician Recruitment Director of Educational Programs Director of Quality Improvement

Table 4–2 The Span of Influence in Project Management and Governance

Span of Influence	Project Management	Governance
Clinical Team	Leader of effort to hire a new team clinician	Team Leader
	Leader of effort to create a team-based peer review process	
Clinical Department	Coordinator of project to create a medical assistant training course for the Ob-Gyn department	Surgery Representative to the Physicians' Council
	Leader of project to design AIDS patient education literature for the internal medicine department	
Geographic Region	Leader of a project to set up a regional urgent care department	Regional Representative to the Physicians' Council
	Leader of project to develop regional CME programs	
Health Care Plan	Leader of quality improvement project to decrease hospital admissions across the plan	Physician Representative of the Plan's Board of Directors
	Leader of project to create a new formulary for pharmaceuticals	

We can also use the span of influence concept to understand the mix of clinical and management responsibilities for physicians in these roles. The larger the span of influence of the position the more time the physician will spend in management and leadership roles, and the less time he or she will spend practicing clinical medicine. For example, the line manager with the smallest span of influence, the team leader, usually spends almost all of his or her time practicing medicine and spends perhaps an hour or two per week on team leadership activities (e.g., organizing and running a team meeting). A medical director, a line manager with a much larger span of influence, usually spends almost all of his or her time in management or leadership roles. Medical directors usually practice medicine less than half of the time and sometimes not at all.

WHAT SKILLS MUST PHYSICIANS ACQUIRE TO BECOME EFFECTIVE LEADERS AND MANAGERS?

Although the role of the physician manager has become more important in our health care system, we are only now starting to identify the core competencies physicians must master to become effective in their new leadership roles. Little formal research is available on this important topic. In 1987 Brown and McCool informally interviewed a wide range of health care leaders (some of whom were physicians) in the hospital setting.[15] They identified a set of common attributes demonstrated by successful medical leaders. These leaders were energetic, hard-working, calm in the face of crises, visionary, and entrepreneurial. They were often described as people-oriented implementers, evaluators, and networkers.

More recently, Ottensmeyer and Key conducted a survey of senior managed care leaders to explore the desirable traits for an effective HMO medical director.[16] These leaders identified communication and interpersonal skills as the most important qualities needed for the role of medical director. Clinical credibility, ego strength, concern about quality, being a "team player," and having a clear philosophy of managed care were other characteristics frequently identified as important for a medical director. Of interest was that the HMO leaders surveyed did not consider formal management training to be very important to the success of medical directors.[17]

Two other surveys illustrated the importance of communication skills. Hartfield surveyed nonphysician supervisors of physician executives and found that frequently, physician managers have the greatest difficulty with communication and time management skills.[17] Another interesting survey by the American College of Physician Executives asked a group of physician managers specifically about communication skills. These managers stated that communication skills were imperative to the success of their organizations. Listening, speaking, and managing conflict were the communication skills rated as most important.[18]

In one of the first articles describing the new role of physician-executive, Hillman et al. took a different view.[4] Looking at the broad set of roles assumed by physician managers in health care, the authors identified a set of traditional management and business subjects that physicians must master to be effective as managers. They suggested that aspiring physician managers undertake formal management training and become knowledgeable about financial analysis, cost-accounting, economics, decision analysis, marketing, and strategic planning.

These studies suggest that effective physician managers must possess various personal characteristics, leadership styles, and technical skills. Which are the key skills or core competencies for physicians looking to undertake management or leadership roles in today's managed care organizations? We asked this question as part of a series of informal interviews with physician managers in selected managed care organizations throughout the country.

The responses were, in many ways, consistent with those of the aforementioned surveys. Most physician managers commented on the importance of having strong clinical skills and credibility. They also identified communication skills as critical to the success of physician managers. The ability to see the "big picture," to create a vision for the organization, and to lead other physicians to develop and accept a common goal or direction were frequently mentioned. Another common theme was the importance of negotiating effectively and the ability to resolve conflicts.

One interesting area of consensus was the lesser importance of technical business skills such as accounting, finance, and marketing. In most managed care organizations, nonphysician managers are usually responsible for these functions. Most physician managers can rely on nonphysician technical experts to assist them in these areas. This diverse group of physician managers clearly saw the "softer" management and leadership skills (e.g., communication, negotiation, developing a vision, teambuilding) as much more important to their success than acquiring and using technical business skills.

The information obtained from our discussions with successful physician managers confirmed our view that a core set of competencies exist that physicians must master to be successful as managers. Furthermore, the traditional clinical training provided in medical schools and residency programs does not teach physicians these skills. These skills and competencies are listed in Exhibit 4–1.

As discussed earlier, a physician's clinical credibility is the foundation upon which he or she builds a management career. Regardless of background or training, physicians interested in management must earn clinical credibility by working as a clinician. In this way, other physicians and health care professionals will gain respect for the physician interested in management. They will also believe that the physician manager really understands their needs as clinicians.

Again, communication skills are fundamental tools for the physician manager. Many physicians are not effective at listening to peers and coworkers, but listening with empathy is a critical step toward establishing an environment of trust between individuals. Speaking clearly, concisely, and with enthusiasm allows the physician manager to engage others in sharing a goal and solving problems. Similarly, effective writing skills enable a manager to communicate ideas to many people simultaneously.

Thus far, we have used the terms *management* and *leadership* somewhat interchangeably. Many books and articles deal extensively with the distinction between managing and leading. Although a detailed discussion of this issue is beyond the scope of

Exhibit 4–1 Key Competencies and Skills for Physician Managers

---

Clinical Credibility

Communication Skills
  Listening
  Speaking
  Writing

Leadership Skills
  Articulating a vision for the future
  Creating an environment of shared responsibility
  Developing the skills of others
  Framing and facilitating critical conversations

Team Building
  Embracing a participatory leadership style
  Developing a common goal or purpose
  Creating a climate of communication and trust
  Effectively leading meetings
  Recognizing and encouraging synergy

Negotiation and Conflict Resolution
  Striving for "win-win" solutions
  Focusing on interests rather than positions
  Encouraging others to communicate and resolve conflict
  Serving as a facilitator

Quality Management
  Articulating a philosophy of continuing improvement
  Embracing the "good apple" approach
  Focusing on processes as the cause of problems
  Empowering the people who do the work to solve problems
  Using data to gain insight into problems

---

this chapter, Kouzes and Posner provide one useful explanation of the difference between leadership and management:

> If there is a clear distinction between the process of managing and leading, it is in the distinction between getting others to do and getting others to want to do. Managers, we believe, get other people to do, but leaders get other people to want to do. Leaders do this by first of all being credible. That is the foundation of leadership. They establish this credibility by their actions—by challenging, inspiring, enabling, modeling, and encouraging.[19]

Burns provides another interesting view of leadership. He says, "Leadership occurs when one or more persons engage with others in such a way that leaders and followers raise one another to higher levels of motivation and morality."[20] For an example of leadership, let's refer back to our fictional HMO, Quality Health-care Plan. Dr. Cathy Chen provided leadership for her clinical team by creating a process by which the team could coordinate their schedules. She then provided encouragement and challenged them to solve the scheduling problem. Ultimately, she facilitated a solution by getting her teammates to work together to create a schedule that met the needs of both the department and the team.

Leadership Styles

In the book *Managing for Excellence*, Bradford and Cohen describe two basic leadership styles.[21] The first and most commonly used style is that of the *heroic leader*. The heroic leader believes his or her role is to make decisions and solve problems. The heroic leader achieves this by being the "expert" on all important topics and always having the final decision. Alternately, the heroic leader will gently convince (or at times coerce) others to do things his or her way. Despite good intentions, the heroic leader creates an environment where people feel powerless, dependent, and uncommitted to the organization's goals.

In contrast, according to Bradford and Cohen, the *postheroic leader* sees his or her role as engaging others in solving problems. The postheroic leader does this by creating an ideal vision of the organization and getting others to share this vision. The postheroic leader develops an environment of shared responsibility for achieving the vision, rather than one in which the leader is solely responsible. Finally, the postheroic leader actively works to develop the talents and skills of others so that individuals and the organization grow and improve.

We strongly believe that postheroic leadership is the optimal style for all leaders—but especially for physician managers. Health care professionals do not respond uniformly to authority

and do not do things just because "the boss says so." They identify with higher principles and goals and want to be part of the
process of solving problems. The postheroic approach has the
potential to tap the wealth of ideas and talents of the clinicians
and staff of managed care organizations. Furthermore, this
approach makes people feel valued and motivated to help the
organization.

Inherent in a postheroic leadership style is the ability to frame
and facilitate critical conversations. This skill involves: (1) articulating clearly the problem or opportunity facing the organization,
department, or team; (2) defining the constraints, boundaries, or
limitations the group must face in solving the problem; and (3)
acting as a facilitator by helping others to communicate, negotiate, and creatively solve the problem.

There are four generic critical conversations physician managers
must facilitate on a recurring basis. These conversations can be
introduced by asking: What is our mission? What are our values?
What expectations do we share? How are we doing? The physician
manager who engages others in these conversations slowly shifts
the responsibility for organizational and personal improvement
from the leader to the larger group. This transformation is critical
to creating an environment of shared responsibility.

Teamwork

Successful physician managers also recognize the importance of
teamwork. Teamwork taps into the creative potential of the group
rather than relying solely on the abilities of the leader. Covey, in his
best-selling book *The Seven Habits of Highly Effective People,* uses the
term *synergy* to describe the potential of a group to achieve more
than the sum of its individual members.[22] Fostering teamwork and
synergy are two of the most crucial skills used by effective leaders.

In their book, *Creating the High Performance Team,* Bucholz and
Roth identify other key elements of building outstanding teams.[23]
They suggest that leaders must actively foster teamwork by
adopting a participatory leadership style. They should work with
teams to develop a common goal or purpose and create a climate
of trust and communication in which teams thrive. Effective leaders empower teams to solve problems and make decisions to

achieve agreed-upon goals. Finally, leaders must be skilled at running meetings. Physician managers who lack this skill are rarely able to build effective teams because their meetings often demotivate and alienate team members.

Conflict Resolution

Another core competency is the ability to resolve conflicts effectively. Physician managers must understand the principles of negotiation. Fischer and Ury, in their popular book *Getting to Yes*, suggest that effective negotiation depends on defining the interests of the individuals in conflict and then creating "win-win" opportunities where both parties get something they want.[24] The effective physician manager can help others to move beyond strategies such as competition or compromise, and help others to see the value of a collaborative approach to conflict resolution. In addition, we believe that effective conflict resolution requires managers to encourage others to resolve their own conflicts. When a conflict arises the skilled manager avoids acting as a judge and instead assumes the role of facilitator.

Quality Enhancement

Finally, physicians in leadership roles must develop competency in the field of quality enhancement. The most popular approach, Total Quality Management (TQM), is a philosophy pioneered by W. Edwards Deming in the 1950s. After his ideas were rejected by American corporations, Deming went to Japan and shared his philosophy with industrial leaders there. The stunning success of Japanese corporations in the automobile and consumer electronics industries in the last 40 years is largely attributed to their commitment to the principles of TQM. Most American corporations are now attempting to become more competitive by adopting the principles of TQM. Similarly, most managed care organizations now recognize the value of TQM and are increasingly using this approach to find ways to deliver high quality health care at a more reasonable cost.

Managers who adhere to the principles of TQM believe that people want to work hard and do a good job. When individuals don't achieve optimal results, these managers look for problems with the processes employees must use to accomplish their work. For example, when a medical assistant repeatedly takes inaccurate blood pressures, the supervisor trained in TQM, rather than blaming the individual, would assume that the medical assistant is doing his or her best. To help the medical assistant improve his or her performance the supervisor will look for "process problems." For instance, the supervisor might ask if the medical assistant received appropriate training. Was the sphygmomanometer malfunctioning? Did the clinician ask the medical assistant to do so many things that he or she had to rush when taking the blood pressure? The manager remains focused on the processes rather than the people as the cause of problems.

Managers who practice TQM strive for continuous improvement. They don't set arbitrary quotas or goals, but insist on slow and steady improvement that continues indefinitely. They achieve these improvements by empowering employees to solve problems and by using data to gain insight into the root causes of problems. They also focus the organization's efforts on meeting the needs of their patients. The following is a real example of how Harvard Community Health Plan (HCHP), a large staff model HMO, took a TQM approach to solve a problem.

Like all HMOs, HCHP is committed to delivering excellent health prevention services to its patients. In the area of screening for breast cancer, HCHP annually performed mammograms on about 70 percent of the women who, according to organization guidelines, should receive this test. Although this screening rate was much better than the national averages, HCHP wanted to do better. The traditional management approach would be to exhort doctors and nurses to pay more attention to breast cancer screening and order more mammograms.

HCHP empowered a team of managers, physicians, nurses, and support staff to study this issue and recommend a strategy to improve mammography screening rates. This team began its work by hypothesizing why some women did not receive mammograms. They then collected data to confirm or dispel their hypothesis. The team found that over 90 percent of women who had an annual comprehensive physical exam in the last two years received a mammogram. On the other hand, less than 40 percent of women who did not have an annual exam received this test. This was surprising, since most of these women made several other visits to their doctor for acute medical problems.

The team then conducted a survey of primary care physicians and nurses and found that these clinicians did not consider it appropriate to raise the issue of breast cancer screening during brief visits for acute problems. Clinicians worried about having the time during these visits to effectively discuss breast cancer screening with women. They also felt uncomfortable ordering a mammogram during a brief visit without having first done a breast examination.

After reviewing these data, the team concluded there were two root causes for suboptimal breast cancer screening. Some women failed to have annual comprehensive examinations, and there was not enough time during acute care visits to educate women about screening and performing breast exams. The team then created a pilot intervention to address these root causes.

At one health center, the team trained medical assistants in primary care to identify from the medical records which women were overdue for mammograms. When one of these women came into the center for an acute medical problem, a medical assistant told her that the doctor recommended that she simultaneously schedule a routine annual examination (including a breast examination) and a mammogram. At the same time, these women were given literature about breast cancer screening guidelines and mammography. They also received a postcard at home reminding them to schedule a physical exam and a mammogram. As a result of these interventions, mammography screening in this one health center rose from 70 percent to 90 percent. There are now plans to adopt this system throughout the rest of Harvard Community Health Plan.

HOW DOES A PHYSICIAN GET STARTED IN MANAGEMENT?

The first step for a physician interested in becoming a physician manager is to acquire the basic skills necessary to be successful in this new role. Some physicians have attempted to do this by enrolling in graduate schools of business or public health and obtaining advanced degrees in business administration (MBA) or health care administration (MPH and MHA). Interestingly, both the previously mentioned survey of HMO medical directors and our own informal survey demonstrate that senior physician managers do not consider an advanced degree to be a necessary qualification for becoming a successful physician manager.

Pros and Cons of the Advanced Degree Strategy

The physician who aspires to become a manager by first obtaining an advanced degree should recognize several disadvantages to this strategy. The course of study required to obtain these degrees usually emphasizes the technical aspects of management such as accounting, marketing, and finance. In many programs, relatively little time is devoted to the core competencies identified earlier in this chapter. It is our experience that successful physician managers always master the "softer" skills of effective communication, participatory leadership, team building, conflict resolution, and quality management. Furthermore, physicians who fail to acquire these competencies are rarely successful in management roles despite their talents in the "hard" management disciplines emphasized in most business and graduate schools.

The second disadvantage is that an advanced degree does not provide young physicians with the clinical credibility they need to be effective leaders in a managed care organization. In the traditional business world, employees respect their managers for their business training. In that setting, an advanced degree is an important credential. In the health care setting, however, physicians and nurses respect their leaders primarily for being excellent clinicians who genuinely understand the challenges and problems of practicing medicine. Without established clinical credibility, a young physician may, in fact, initially find an advanced degree to be a disadvantage—peers may view the young physician manager as "one of them" rather than as a fellow clinician.

Finally, and perhaps most importantly, there is the problem of cost. Full-time tuition for advanced degree programs can be extremely high and is probably prohibitive for most young physicians who have already acquired large debts to finance their medical training. Few young doctors will find it possible to give up their practice income for the one or more years required by these programs. As an alternative, some business or public health schools offer courses on evenings and weekends that can lead to advanced degrees. This option makes it possible to spread the costs of an advanced degree over more years and permits a physician to continue to practice medicine while studying on nights and weekends. Although this approach is financially more attractive, adding the rigors of graduate school study to the demands of a busy clinical practice is often unrealistic and exhausting.

Despite these limitations and obstacles, an advanced degree can be a significant asset for the motivated individual. Most degree programs introduce physicians to a wide range of important business and health care management concepts not usually taught in medical schools or residency programs (e.g., legal aspects of health care delivery, medical ethics, information system management, marketing principles, data analysis, and statistics). In addition, the advanced degree can be a powerful credential that distinguishes an individual as a "professional physician manager." Finally, some degree programs are now developing courses to teach many of the core competencies discussed earlier in this chapter.

Growth Opportunities

Another—and for many physicians—more practical approach to acquiring key management skills and competencies is to participate in progressively more challenging management roles within their current setting or institution. This strategy provides the opportunity for acquiring clinical credibility by working primarily as a clinician while simultaneously developing the core competencies needed to succeed as a physician manager.

For example, a resident could initially volunteer to be on the hospital's medical education committee or participate on the intern selection committee. This would provide an opportunity to observe and develop good communication, teamwork, and negotiation skills. If successful in these early management roles, the resident would probably have the opportunity to serve on other committees or task forces and acquire higher level skills. Some residents may have the opportunity to become chief resident and develop additional leadership skills.

Similarly, a physician in private practice contemplating a future management career in managed care has similar opportunities. He or she can also volunteer for hospital committees. Alternately, serving in the role of "office manager" for the office's support staff would enable a physician to practice communication, negotiating, teambuilding, and leadership skills.

A physician currently working in a managed care plan has many opportunities to develop management and leadership skills. Volunteering for committees and task forces within the organization is a useful approach. Participation in national managed care organizations such as the National Association of Managed Care Physicians (NAMCP) or the Group Health Association of America (GHAA) provides additional opportunities for physicians to learn more about managed care and acquire leadership skills.

Many clinical departments have "team leader" roles that offer an excellent opportunity for physicians to develop and practice the key skills of leadership. Considering the scarcity of highly competent physician managers, success at these early management experiences will usually lead to opportunities to head a committee or project. Eventually, physicians who demonstrate competency in these skills and an interest in leadership activities will be offered a more formal management role, such as chief of a department.

Finally, there are an infinite number of opportunities for physicians to develop leadership skills in nonmedical organizations. Most organizations welcome the participation of an energetic physician. For example, the aspiring physician manager could serve on a school board or volunteer for a local government committee. After mastering some of these competencies, physicians have a much better chance at succeeding in their first leadership roles within their health care organizations.

In any of these early management experiences, physicians must not limit their approach to trial and error. Unless they find other ways to acquire critical skills, many physicians will have difficulty with their early management experiences and become demotivated and disillusioned. In our experience, physicians are much more likely to achieve success and enjoyment in early management roles if they have selected an experienced physician manager to serve as their mentor.

The Value of a Mentor

The mentor serves as a resource for the physician as he or she faces new management problems or challenges. The mentor can suggest approaches that help the physician avoid critical management mistakes. The mentor will also provide the new physician manager with crucial support and encouragement. For an example, let's return for a moment to our mythical HMO, Quality Healthcare Plan. Dr. Bob Bright is a gynecologist who volunteers to chair a committee created to recommend whether the department should buy a new ultrasound machine. He has trouble running the first few committee meetings. Committee members arrive late, frequently interrupt each other, and stray from the agenda. The group fails to reach any conclusions and Dr. Bright becomes frustrated.

He decides to ask his department chief for advice. After listening to Dr. Bright's account of the meetings, the chief makes a few suggestions. Dr. Bright should set some ground rules for the meetings. The chief suggests that Dr. Bright ask the group to set the ground rules and then follow them. At the next meeting, Dr. Bright points out to his committee that the meetings have not gone well. He asks the group for some ideas for ground rules. One member suggests that everyone should arrive on time. Another suggests that Dr. Bright recognize people before they speak. A third member volunteers that someone should distribute an agenda before the meeting. Dr. Bright recommends that the group commit to following these rules and agrees to distribute the agendas himself.

At the next meeting, everyone arrives on time. Dr. Bright writes the ground rules on the blackboard at the front of the room. He reviews the rules and reminds the group that they agreed to abide by them. Dr. Bright reviews the agenda he distributed a week before the meeting. He then invites discussion of the first topic. Soon, someone interrupts while another committee member is speaking. Dr. Bright gently reminds the group of the ground rule that states that he must recognize members before they speak. The discussion continues and the group systematically works through the agenda. As the meeting ends, the group and Dr. Bright are pleased that they made real progress toward reaching a decision on whether to buy the new piece of equipment.

Continuing Education

Besides acquiring management skills through progressive experiences and selecting a mentor, physicians interested in management can take continuing education courses designed for physician managers. The American College of Physician Executives, a rapidly growing organization committed to promoting the role of physician manager, offers a series of continuing education courses specifically designed to introduce physicians to important concepts in health care management. Physicians who already work for a managed care organization can often take advantage of management programs offered by their health care plans. Finally, physicians may choose to take selected management courses from a local university or graduate school without investing the time and money needed to pursue an advanced degree.

Another important strategy for acquiring management and leadership skills is to develop a program for ongoing self-education. There is a plethora of books on management and leadership topics in virtually every library and bookstore. Many books offer useful insights and approaches to management that physicians can apply successfully in managed care settings. Keeping in mind the set of key competencies outlined earlier, physicians should seek out books about leadership styles, teambuilding, conflict resolution, negotiation, and quality management. Since the successful physician manager is committed to a lifelong program of self-education, he or she has usually read many books on these topics. Experienced physician managers are often a valuable resource for the physician looking for good "management tips."

In summary, there are two basic approaches available to the aspiring physician manager. For the small number of physicians who have the time, financial resources, and commitment, pursuing an advanced degree in management or health care administration is an approach that can lead to a satisfying job as a physician manager within a managed care organization. Nonetheless, our experiences suggest that prior to enrolling in a course of graduate study, it is critical that physicians carefully establish clinical credibility by working as a clinician within a managed care organization. Also, they should choose advanced degree programs with a good selection of courses that address the core competencies discussed in this chapter.

The second—and for most physicians—more practical approach to acquiring management and leadership expertise is by undertaking progressively more challenging management experiences within their residency programs, group practices, hospitals, or managed care organizations. Physicians also should select a mentor to accelerate the learning process and provide necessary support and encouragement. Finally, physicians can develop a program of ongoing self-education in management by attending continuing education courses and reading about leadership and management in books and journals.

CONCLUSION

Considering the growing consensus about the problems inherent in our health care system, managed care organizations will certainly play a key role in this nation's efforts to deliver high quality medical care at an affordable cost to its population. Unless our country adopts a government-financed and managed national health care system such as the one in Great Britain (which our population strongly opposes), it seems inevitable that managed care will continue to grow and prosper.

In fact, the most popular current strategy for restraining the growth of national health care expenditures is called *managed competition*. Its architects suggest that the entire U.S. population be enrolled in managed care plans that compete with each other in terms of both the cost and quality of the health care they deliver.[3] The current administration is advocating managed competition as a model for reforming health care. We believe that the political environment will fuel the continued growth of managed care over the next five to ten years.

This growth means that managed care organizations will need many more physician managers. These organizations recognize that the challenging task of providing excellent health care while controlling costs requires a partnership of clinicians and management. Managed care organizations must therefore recruit and train more good physician managers if they are to grow and be successful. Many of these organizations are already finding it very difficult to hire or develop good physician managers to fill important roles within their health care plans. The number of opportunities for physicians interested in management will increase dramatically within managed care organizations over the next decade.

Not only will the number of opportunities increase, but it is our belief that the role of physician manager also will evolve. The current dominant model of physician managers supervising other clinicians in a hierarchical structure will be replaced by physician *leaders* who facilitate "self-managing" teams of clinicians and staff. Physician leaders will do this by helping clinicians and teams develop their own competencies in the areas of communication, teamwork, conflict resolution, and quality management. Physician managers will become teachers and facilitators rather than bosses and supervisors.

Physician managers of the future will also be charged with fostering the creation of a vision for the future for managed care organizations and encouraging clinician "buy-in" to this vision. Managed care organizations face a tremendous challenge in their efforts to minimize costs in an environment where the population is aging, expensive technologies are created almost daily, and Americans expect unlimited access to health care services. Physician leaders have a pivotal role to play in helping their organizations find ways to face these challenges. Not least, they must forge a partnership between managers, clinicians, and patients in order to arrive at reasonable compromises—those that promise optimal use of our limited resources and enhanced quality of patient care.

REFERENCES

1. Guthrie M. Why physicians move into management. In: Wesley C, ed. *New Leadership in Health Care Management: The Physician Executive.* Tampa, Fla: American College of Physician Executives; 1988.

2. Ottensmeyer DJ, Key MK. Managed health care: the benefits approach to cost and quality. *Personnel.* 1990;67(9):29–30, 32.

3. Enthoven A, Kronick R. A consumer-choice health plan for the 1990s. Universal health insurance in a system designed to promote quality and economy. *N Engl J Med.* 1989;320 :29-37.

4. Hillman AL, Nash DB, Kissick WL, Martin SP. Managing the medical-industrial complex. *N Engl J Med.* 1985;315:511–1315

5. Kindig DA, Lastiri S. Administrative medicine: a new medical specialty? *Health Affairs.* Winter 1986:146–156.

6. Nash DB. The physician executive: part 1, growing demand for an emerging Subspecialty. *Consultant.* 1987;27:97–108.

7. Doyne M. Physicians as managers. *Healthcare Forum Journal.* September/October 1987:11–13.

8. Schneller ES. The leadership and executive potential of physicians in an era of managed care systems. *Hospital and Health Services Administration.* 1991;36:43–55.

9. Nash DB, Hillman AL. Physician–executives can be mediators. *Modern Healthcare.* November 21,1986:49.

10. Raelin JA. *The Clash of Cultures: Managers and Professionals.* Boston, Mass: Harvard Business School Press; 1991.

11. Brook RH, Park RE, Chassin MR, Solomon DH, Keesey J, Kossecoff J. Predicting the appropriate use of carotid endarterectomy, upper gastrointestinal endoscopy, and coronary angiography." *N Engl J Med.* 1990;323:1173–1177.

12. Winslow CM, Kosecoff JB, Chassin M, Kanouse DE, Brook RH. The appropriateness of coronary artery bypass surgery. *JAMA.* 1988;260:505–509.

13. Winslow CM, Solomon DH, Chassin MR, Kosecoff J, Merrick NJ, Brook RH. The appropriateness of carotid endarterectomy. *N Engl J Med.* 1988;318:721–727.

14. Hillman AL Managing the physician: rules versus incentives. *Health Affairs;* Winter 1991:138–146.

15. Brown M, McCool BP. "High-performing managers: leadership attributes for the 1990s. *Health Care Management Review.* 1987;12:69–75.

16. Ottensmeyer DJ, Key MK. Lessons learned hiring HMO medical directors. *Health Care Management Review.*1991;16:21–30.

17. Hartfield JE. Physicians in management: the costs, challenges, and rewards. In: *The Physician Executive.* Tampa, Fla: American College of Physician Executives; 1988.

18. Staley SS, Staley CS. Physician executives and communication. *Physician Executive.* 1989;15:15–17.

19. Kouzes JM, Posner BZ. *The Leadership Challenge.* San Francisco, CA:Jossey-Bass Publishers; 1987: 27.

20. Burns JM. *Leadership.* New York: Harper & Row; 1978:20.

21. Bradford D, Cohen A. *Managing for Excellence.* New York: John Wiley & Sons; 1984.

22. Covey SR. *The Seven Habits of Highly Effective People.* New York: Simon & Schuster; 1990.

23. Bucholz S, Roth T. *Creating the High Performance Team.* New York: John Wiley & Sons; 1987.

24. Fischer R, Ury W. *Getting to Yes.* New York: Penguin Books; 1981.

Editorial Commentary

Susan L. Howell

David B. Nash

Most students enter medical school because they want to practice medicine. Beyond clinical practice, the physician's career choices have traditionally been defined within the realm of teaching and research. As physicians are increasingly called upon to assume leadership positions within the managed care field, a new career path is fast emerging: that of the physician manager.

Harry L. Leider and Marc A. Bard describe this burgeoning career track for physicians who are interested in medical management within the managed care arena. Dr. Leider is a medical director at the Harvard Community Health Plan, one of the nation's preeminent prepaid group practices, and is a former Robert Wood Johnson Clinical Scholar from the University of Washington in Seattle. Dr. Bard is Director of Medical Staff Development at Harvard Community Health Plan and Principle of Marc Bard Management Consultants.

Doctors Leider and Bard offer a comprehensive account of the types of management and leadership roles available to physicians in managed care. They discuss how the managed care setting in particular holds a potential wealth of opportunities for those who wish to be agents of change at both the clinical and executive levels. They also offer practical advice regarding breaking into the field, including the skills, leadership styles, and personality characteristics that are requisites for the successful physician manager; the pursuit of an advanced degree or targeted courses offered through professional organizations such as the American College of Physician Executives; and the value of having a mentor.

Until recently, the majority of physicians who assumed management responsibilities invariably did so coincidentally and were perceived by their colleagues as shirking the rigors of clinical practice. Prevailing attitudes toward physician managers have changed markedly, however, due in large part to managed care's relatively newfound acceptance and the knowledge that the managed care structure necessitates a close partnership between clinicians and management. Medical schools and other educational programs are responding, and today clinicians are choosing careers in management in growing numbers. Drs. Leider and Bard explain this phenomenon, citing a major national survey of physician managers, and informal interviews conducted by them and their staff. The responses are inspiring and shed further light on this new breed of physician.

Dr. Leider's position as a line manager and Dr. Bard's position in program management makes them well-equipped to forecast the future role of physician managers in HMOs. As this newfound specialty continues to strive for professional legitimization, its impact will be profoundly felt at all levels of the health care system. As liaisons, management information specialists, advocates, administrators, strategic planners, clinicians, and leaders, the managed care physician executive brings activism and pragmatism to today's health care system.

Chapter 5

The National Association of Managed Care Physicians

William C. Williams III
R.S. Venable
Daniel H. Friend

INTRODUCTION

Today's health care system is complex and confusing. Health care costs are out of control, according to President Clinton at his December 1992 economic summit in Little Rock, Arkansas, just prior to taking office. By the end of the decade, the United States is expected to spend $1.6 trillion for health care.[1] Yet, nearly 37 million Americans currently have no health care coverage. Consequently, strategies continue to evolve to assure economical access to quality health care for all Americans.

That's where managed health care comes in. Managed health care is the practice of managing the health care dollar to get the most care for the money. From the patient's perspective, that means getting quality care. From the industry's point of view, managing those dollars is accomplished through the establishment of organizational models such as health maintenance organizations (HMOs), preferred provider organizations (PPOs), exclusive provider arrangements (EPAs), and point of service (POS) plans. (See Exhibit 5–1.)

This chapter will briefly summarize developments in American health care that led to the formation of managed care approaches and the National Association of Managed Care Physicians (NAMCP). We will explore the existing forms of managed care and then discuss the innovative approach taken by a group of doctors who banded together to further optimize these managed care models in favor of optimal quality medical care for American patients.

Exhibit 5–1 Managed Care Megatrends

---

1. Managed care alternative health plans will become dominant by approximately 1994 (50 percent national enrollment).

2. The "insurance" concept is obsolete and insurers are rapidly repositioning themselves as PPOs.

3. PPOs have surpassed HMOs in national enrollment and will continue to exceed HMO membership in the 1990s.

4. HMOs and PPOs will blend into managed care plans with multiple buyer options, shared control systems, and interlocking provider networks.

5. All areas and populations will come to accept managed care in the next three years. The PPO concept will be flexibly adapted to distinct local populations and consumer preferences, and third-party administrators will make managed care options available to small employers.

6. Major purchasers (employers, unions, government) will cut out the middlemen (HMOs, PPOs, insurance companies) and create their own buyer-managed systems.

7. For the poor and medically uninsured, local and state governments may turn to managed care to provide the solution to ever-increasing expenditures and cost control; state and local governments may begin to phase out public hospitals, preferring to contract out to HMOs and PPOs or to a selected network of local providers.

8. Medicare beneficiaries may rapidly abandon fee-for-service in favor of Medicare HMOs and PPOs that coordinate benefits, eliminate out-of-pocket costs, and provide low-cost drug benefits.

9. Managed care minimarkets, such as behavioral health, Workers' Compensation, and occupational medicine, will become increasingly profitable and competitive. Case management, provider risk sharing, and strict control of inpatient care will characterize these new arrangements.

10. Inpatient care, the traditional business base of health care, will be further eroded as managed care expands. Expect admissions, patient days, and length of stay to fall further until hospital use rates reach 400 days per 1,000 persons by 1995.

Source: Adapted from *The New Medicine: Reshaping Medical Practice and Health Care Management,* by Russell C. Coile, Jr., p. 134, © 1990 Aspen Publishers, Inc.

The Managed Care System: A Definition

A managed care health plan is a combination of interdependent systems that include the financing and delivery of health care services. More specifically, managed health care plans utilize the following elements: (1) arrangements with selected providers to furnish a comprehensive set of health care services to members, (2) explicit standards for the selection of health care providers, (3) programs for ongoing quality assurance and utilization review, and (4) financial incentives for members to use providers and procedures associated with the plan.[2]

History of Managed Care

Forms of what today are called prepaid plans were established in the last century. Their goal was to help meet the health care needs of potentially underserved groups such as those in rural areas and in the lumber, mining, and railroad industries. In urban areas, such groups often provided for the health care of members or charges of benevolent societies.

By the 20th century, there was a broadening of the kinds of managed care provided by health care plans. For example, Dr. Michael Shadid started a rural farmers' cooperative health plan in Elk City, Oklahoma, in 1929. In that same year, Donald Ross and Clifford Loos, two Los Angeles physicians, established a doctor-owned and controlled group practice prepayment plan to provide 2,000 water company employees with health services.

By the 1930s and 1940s, businesses and industries became interested in prepaid health plans. Some of these models were precursors to the modern HMO: (1) Group Health Plan Association in Washington, DC, 1937; (2) Kaiser-Permanente Medical Care Programs, 1942; (3) Group Health Cooperative of Puget Sound in Seattle, Washington; and (4) Health Insurance Plan of Greater New York, 1947.

Starting in the Eisenhower administration, policymakers began to look at prepaid health plans as an alternative to traditional fee-for-service care. Medicare was planned in the late 1950s and implemented in 1966 as a federal form of prepaid care. This was primarily because fee-for-service systems provided incentives that contributed to the already escalating costs of health care. However, Medicare soon ran into financial trouble because medical providers were "incentivized" to bill more services in the face of declining reimbursement per service.

In response to these cost concerns, the Nixon administration in the 1970s began to look at *health maintenance organizations*— a term coined by Paul M. Ellwood, a Minneapolis physician and former director of the American Rehabilitation Foundation. HMOs were touted as a friendlier form of control than national health insurance.

In 1973, Congress passed the Health Maintenance Organization Act. The legislation "provided grants to support the development of HMOs in various geographic regions, preempted restrictive state laws, required employers to offer federally qualified HMOs and set standards for federal qualification of HMOs."[2] The act served as a stimulus for HMO development and led to experimentation in health care delivery. Many of these activities led the way to what is known today as managed care. Gatekeeping, utilization controls, and quality assessment and review were concepts introduced in early forms of managed care. With 1976 and 1978 amendments lessening federal qualification requirements, more federal funds became available. Between 1973 and 1983, the U.S. Government provided $145 million in grants and $219 million in loans to establish 115 HMOs. Between 1974 and 1980, nonfederal entities invested $253 million to form HMOs.[3]

HOW HMOs WORK

Early HMOs were developed around major medical groups. Some larger HMO programs, such as Kaiser-Permanente Health Plan and the Group Health Cooperative of Puget Sound, at one time owned or controlled their own hospitals. Today's HMO functions as more of a service broker, contracting with hospitals and a network of physicians organized as independent provider associations or medical staff groups.

Despite many variations on the method of medical care delivery, all HMOs function in a similar federally regulated framework.[4] The HMO assumes financial risk for providing health care. It both ensures and arranges for health care delivery. This method contrasts with that of traditional indemnity insurance plans, which act as a fiscal go-between for the payers of health care services, such as employers and individual subscribers, and the fee-for-service sector that provides these health care services for patients.

The HMO has a well-defined population of patients. An employer group usually enrolls its employees (the patients) in the HMO for a set period of time. This contrasts with the patient population of individual physicians, who typically serve ill-defined groups of individuals who come and go at will. It offers voluntary participation by patients. Employers usually offer HMOs as one choice, along with indemnity and PPO options. The decision to offer a particular health care plan is made by the employer.

HMOs deal with a defined and restricted provider panel composed of health care professionals and facilities. Physicians and other health care providers agree to participate on the financial basis of a discount from usual and customary fee-for-service costs. Although actual fees per service may be the same as private practice, the number of services approved is much lower than traditional private practice because specialty testing and evaluation are reviewed by utilization representatives of the health plan. Medically unnecessary services are not usually provided.

Methods of Quality Assurance

HMOs use various techniques to ensure that the quality of care they provide is as good, if not better, than that of the more traditional forms of health care delivery. Techniques to assure enrollees quality and customer satisfaction include grievance procedures, satisfaction surveys, advisory committees, and scrutinizing utilization and outcome data. Physicians are carefully screened before being credentialed. Their care is under periodic physician peer review. Education and/or suspension from the plan is recommended when there is recurrent evidence of suboptimal care.[2] HMOs use utilization review to ensure that enrollees are provided with appropriate medical services. Utilization review is a collective term for the following activities:[2]

1. *Precertification:* Prior to elective hospitalizations, surgical procedures, and certain diagnostic tests, evaluations are conducted against standard criteria for appropriateness before payment is authorized.
2. *Concurrent Review:* This procedure is the formal review of
continuing hospitalizations to determine whether the length
of stay and any subsequent medical intervention is appropriate and consistent with good medical practice.
3. *Discharge Planning:* To minimize length of hospital stay, the
HMO arranges in advance for care to be received after the
patient is discharged.
4. *Case Management:* Systematic reviews are conducted to identify patients who, because of the severity of illness or intensity
of service needed, are likely to require protracted hospitalization or intensive therapy. These patients are tracked to ensure
that they receive the most appropriate and cost-effective care.

Claims review and retrospective review are not part of utilization review, but they are ways to assure quality. An HMO will
review claims for enrollee eligibility, appropriateness of service,
proper billing, and appropriateness of referral. In retrospective
review, the HMO looks at claims and encounter referral data to
compare actual utilization against what was expected. This study
reveals physician practice patterns, which can then be evaluated
against norms to determine physician efficiency. This practice of
physician profiling is useful in measuring and assessing quality.

OTHER FORMS OF MANAGED CARE

In HMOs, there is a fiscal intermediary representing the patient,
largely on behalf of the employer, in the interest of saving money.
Other forms of managed care emerge as intermediaries change
between patient/doctor and the employer.

PPOs are a mixture of the traditional fee-for-service indemnity
insurance plans and HMOs. Like HMOs, PPOs are organized networks of hospitals and physicians. But unlike HMOs, PPOs do
not contract for full responsibility to provide certain services.

Rather, PPOs serve as service brokers to insurance companies, employers, the government, third-party intermediaries, and other major buyers. A PPO negotiates with hospitals and physicians a price for services at a discounted rate. PPO enrollees may choose a preferred provider from the PPO network. The incentive for the enrollees is full payment for services when services are provided by a preferred source. If they use nonpreferred providers, the consumer is responsible for a certain percentage of copayments.

EPAs, an experimental offshoot of PPOs, bring buyers and sellers of health care closer together. This trend to cut out middle organizations such as health insurers (including HMOs) and third-party administrators is yet another method that may help control increasing costs. As major employers become increasingly comfortable as informed health care purchasers, they typically begin to select their own network of preferred hospitals and physicians. Employers often use the company health plan to channel employees to providers selected by the company for company-determined services. With fewer administrative costs, there is usually more money for a broader array of covered benefits and services for employees, and even additional benefits such as well-child care and health promotion services offered at no extra cost.

For the employer, cost control is the largest incentive of EPAs. Pricing can be set using experience rating—the employer's experience—rather than community rating, which reflects the overall pattern of health use. A company-sponsored EPA, also known as a negotiated provider arrangement, lets the company obtain the lowest prices from providers selected by the company for cost, quality, and location. The company is also allowed to tailor the package of covered services based on the employer's experience.

Point-of-Service (POS) plans offer a combination of features found in the HMO and the PPO. The concept was first developed by HMOs to give enrollees more choices. The POS plan allows enrollees, at the time of service, to decide whether to use an HMO or PPO system for health care. Although the HMO structure prevails, the POS enrollee may use out-of-network providers. However, this choice will result in higher enrollee copayments to these outside providers.

The POS plan that uses the HMO network also has similar contracting arrangements. Less common is the point of service plan that uses the PPO's traditional discounted fee-for-service arrangement. The PPO providers do not share in the risk for out-of-network care, and the enrollee is the only one with financial incentive for getting care within the network. However, there is a defined provider network in both the HMO- and PPO-based POS plans.

Despite differences in payment methods and coverage, all of the managed care alternatives to the traditional HMO work to assure quality care for minimal cost. Utilization controls are not as rigorous in non-HMO plans but costs are usually higher. There are fewer quality improvement opportunities in non-HMO settings. However, the overall care provided in all systems is relatively uniform, largely due to the current regulatory and malpractice environment experienced by physicians and hospitals in everyday business.

THE FORMATION OF THE NATIONAL ASSOCIATION OF MANAGED CARE PHYSICIANS

The National Association of Managed Care Physicians (NAMCP) was founded in 1991 to give managed care physicians a voice. It is the only association organized primarily to serve the needs of this growing group of physicians, who number over 360,000 of the nearly 6,000,000 licensed physicians in America.

Physicians directly affect 85 percent of the near trillion-dollar expense portion of the health care cost equation through providing direct medical services to patients, ordering X-rays, lab work and prescriptions, and admitting patients to hospitals. This amounts annually to hundreds of billions of dollars. Yet, health care decisions are made daily by professional administrators, financial officers, corporate benefits managers, public officials, and politicians—parties with no medical training and no personal obligation to the welfare of patients. Very often, input from the front lines of medical delivery—the practicing physician—is absent. The voice of the physician, who is legally, ethically, and morally responsible for direct patient care, must be raised in a proactive and positive manner to affect managed health care delivery. Physicians provide the patient advocacy and a quality of care perspective that cannot be achieved through input by any other party in health care. Positive involvement by physicians in managed health care can ensure continuous improvement in the quality of health care services.

NAMCP Mission and Vision Statements

The NAMCP was incorporated as a nonprofit 501(c)6 association in January 1991 by W.C. Williams III, MD, a Richmond, Virginia, managed health care physician with more than ten years' family practice experience. The NAMCP was formed to educate physicians about responsible resource allocation and to give them an input at all levels of involvement in the managed care arena. The NAMCP provides a forum for practicing physicians to communicate their concerns about the changing health care environment.

The mission of the NAMCP is to enhance the ability of practicing physicians to proactively participate within the managed health care arena through research, communication, and education. It is dedicated to advancing the professional and personal development of its members and to maintain quality health care in the managed health care industry.

The association supports the following:

1. Employer, patient, and physician education and stronger physician-patient relationships in managed health care
2. Physician participation in the development of practice criteria, pertinent quality assurance, and appropriate utilization management criteria; and in all regulation and legislation affecting physicians in managed health care
3. An information network and clearinghouse for physicians in the managed health care industry
4. A variety of programs to promote communications among managed health care physicians and other health care professionals, including academia; government; the pharmaceutical industry; insurance carriers; employers; unions; other profes-

sional associations; and the management of managed health care organizations

5. Public awareness of the costs and benefits of appropriate medical care services in a managed health care system

NAMCP Objectives

The NAMCP has established objectives that are divided into two categories: professional practice issues and regulatory and legislative issues. Each category falls under the rubric of furthering the education of physicians in the tools and skills necessary to flourish in today's health care arena

The NAMCP is carrying out its objectives in several ways. First, it strives to disseminate current clinical information and research via affiliation with current texts, the member newsletter, NAMCP bi-monthly professional journal, and reviews through U.S. HealthLink, a national data company. Second, it seeks affiliation with other health care-related entities through cosponsorships and joint projects. Current project partners include:

- National Managed Health Care Congress
- American Hospital Association
- Individual Case Management Association
- National Health Lawyers Association
- National College of Medical Quality

Third, it sponsors its own quarterly regional conferences, whose focus is broadly medico-legal, and specifically, business- and clinically focused; and an annual communications seminar, which seeks to enhance physician-patient and physician-health professional relationships. The topics of two of the NAMCP's 1993 quarterly conferences were health care reform and health care in the 1990s.

Physician Education Programs

The NAMCP is also in the process of developing both a school and an institute for managed care. Initially, course material will be aimed at medical directors, utilizing the association's affiliation with the Kellogg School of Business of Northwestern University in Chicago. This school will be expanded to provide regional educational programs for all physicians. It will lead toward the development of a managed care credentialing body, and provide primary verification for all physicians working within managed care environments.

A managed health care curriculum for medical schools is currently being developed for future physicians. The goal is to inform them about key terms and concepts and provide them with an overview of managed care. This will allow them to become informed and proactive from a managed care standpoint early in their careers. The first programs in medical schools started at the University of South Florida in Tampa in July 1993, with a medical student rotation in managed care for fourth-year students.

In affiliation with a national information company, the NAMCP will develop a resume database and placement referral service for physicians. This will expedite placement and credentialing of physicians in both primary and specialty care for managed care plans across America.

Legislative Issues

Since regulatory and legislative issues abound in the daily practice of medicine, the NAMCP will provide timely review and advice on legislation affecting physicians in the managed health care industry. It will participate in the development of pertinent quality assurance and appropriate utilization management criteria, and the regulatory guidelines that may impact these areas. To this end, the NAMCP has been involved with the Clinton administration since December 1992, providing advice and counsel during the health care reform initiatives ultimately chaired by Hillary Rodham Clinton.

To facilitate these governmental objectives, the NAMCP, established as a nonprofit lobbying organization, employs a lobbyist in Washington, DC, who serves as a link between the association and Capitol Hill. Consequently, the association is working to become a recognized voice on matters that affect doctors in the managed health care setting.

Membership

Associations continually seek to expand their membership, and the NAMCP is no exception. From its inception in 1991, the NAMCP has grown to nearly 12,000 members as of this writing.

The organization, which holds its annual meeting in the spring, offers two types of memberships, individual and corporate. There are four different kinds of individual memberships with varying membership dues structures:

1. *Regular:* Any licensed physician, MD or DO. This category represents the only voting membership category of the association
2. *Associate:* Any allied health professional who is an employee of a managed health care system—for example, nurse practitioners, physician assistants, etc.
3. *Resident or Student:* Any resident or student presently enrolled in an accredited residency program or medical school who has an interest in managed health care.
4. *Other:* All other interested individuals not meeting above membership criteria but who have an interest in managed health care from a personal or business perspective.

Corporate memberships include various levels and types of business entities or agencies that provide services or goods to the managed health care industry. Corporate members include consultants and industry-related firms, pharmaceutical firms, hospitals, managed care plans and organizations, and other physician and health care-related associations.

The NAMCP also has advisory boards and panels comprised of physician members as well as representatives from the major health insurance carriers; national and regional managed health care plans; the pharmaceutical industry; the hospital industry; and employer/health benefits administrator industry.

The organization's officers and directors are nominated by the board of directors. Actual administration and most services such as marketing, direct mail, publishing, and list management are provided through experienced professionals in the NAMCP national offices in Richmond, Virginia and in the Western Region office in San Francisco, California.

Volunteer Committees. Volunteer committees play an important role in the development of an organization and in helping it realize its objectives. While associations can rely on professional management for administrative purposes, the core direction and substance comes from the membership.

Committees provide an organized means of constructively channeling member involvement. They also serve to identify and encourage new leaders and directions for the association.

The chairperson for each committee is nominated from the actual or potential membership and professional outside advisors from appropriate businesses. Committee size ranges, on the average, from eight to fifteen members.

Each committee receives administrative support to maintain the productivity and interest of chairpersons and advisors who have heavy demands on their time. There is no set schedule for the committees; instead, each group meets on an as-needed basis.

The NAMCP has formed five initial committees. They include: Membership, Education, Publications, Medical Directors and Utilization Management, and Quality Assurance. The NAMCP plans to form a total of 17 volunteer committees. The long-term association's plan includes the following committees:

- *Membership:* Includes all aspects of the membership growth of the organization, including the marketing and member benefit development efforts. Regional membership committees are planned for 1993 to develop state chapters and liaisons for 1994.
- *Membership Services and Communications:* Responsible for all regular ongoing communications with the membership including telephone support, regular mailing, and the newsletter.
- *Regulatory and Legislative Issues:* Involved with formulating and promoting the association's interests in regulatory, legislative, and health care policy areas. Especially responsible for the lobbying efforts of the association.
- *Utilization Management and Quality Assurance:* Responsible for the development of pertinent utilization management and quality assurance criteria and related issues.
- *Practice Criteria:* Responsible for the development of practice criteria and related issues.

- *Education:* Responsible for developing continuing education programs for members, including CME credit and the development of NAMCP physician credentialing for managed health care professionals.
- *Professional Association Liaison:* Responsible for close communications with all major professional associations.
- *Industry Liaison:* Responsible for programs and relations with industry firms such as employers, pharmaceutical companies, medical equipment suppliers, insurers, home health providers, and others.
- *Public Relations:* Responsible for developing broader public relations efforts including a regular ongoing press relations program, as well as press releases in response to specific issues. This committee is also responsible for ongoing relations with appropriate medical publishers and the broadcast media.
- *Publications:* Responsible for more complex, longer-term publishing projects such as journals, magazines, and monograph series on subjects of interest to the membership base. More routine publications, such as the newsletter, will be handled by the membership services and education committees.
- *Research:* Responsible for all research-related issues including gathering relevant information for the membership, and commissioning and managing the association's own research.
- *Finance:* Responsible for both financial oversight and long-range financial stability of the association.
- *Meetings:* Responsible for the program content of NAMCP meetings as well as displaying information about the organization at the meetings of other associations.
- *NAMCP Foundation:* In some cases, the funding and management of educational grants requires a separate educational foundation affiliated with, but distinct from, the NAMCP. This committee will work toward establishing the needs of the health care industry and finding and overseeing the funding of each specific project.
- *State Chapter Liasion:* Responsible for helping to develop and support state chapters of the association. The state chapters of the various state medical societies can serve as models for this committee.

- *Technology Assessment:* Responsible for communicating the evaluation and accommodation of technology in managed care settings.
- *Medical Director:* Responsible for the unique needs of medical directors, including regular communications with the NAMCP.

The Future of the NAMCP

If present trends continue, there will be more than 40 million Americans enrolled in HMOs in 1993. Other forms of managed care plans (PPOs, POS plans, EPAs, Physician-Hospital Organizations) coupled with health care reform will cover over 200 million Americans by 1995. As a result, the NAMCP's future is bright as a proactive force encouraging education and physician input in managed care.

To further enhance its future utility to practicing physicians, NAMCP has or is in the process of establishing several programs. The association currently publishes a newsletter to give regular, pertinent updates about issues that involve physicians in managed health care. This will be expanded to provide more frequent updates as needed to keep pace with changes in the American medical delivery system.

The NAMCP's bimonthly managed care journal was released in Summer 1993. Among the topics covered: clinical research information such as studies and reviews; drug information and updates; personal finance information; industry activity and changes; continuing medical education information; and health care and business management information. Also featured are academically referred clinical application articles. Medico-legal and regulatory updates and analysis are included on a regular basis. A Tips and Techniques section is provided to empower physicians to optimize their involvement in the changing medical practice environment of the 1990s and beyond.

The NAMCP information network database coordinates a broad variety of clinical research studies, including those funded by pharmaceutical companies, the government, and managed health care systems. It will be on-line in Fall 1993.

There is currently a toll-free number (1–800–722–0376) that serves as a clearinghouse for information on any issue of concern to physicians dealing with managed health care systems. This service refers members to the appropriate sources rather than duplicates information sources.

Projects scheduled for late 1993 and into 1994 include the development of:

- appropriate utilization management and quality assurance systems for the managed health care industry
- appropriate practice criteria for the managed health care industry
- library and resource center for providing access to the world of managed care literature for physicians and others interested in managed care
- relationships with other associations and organizations to coordinate the efficient and effective referral of inquiries on managed care topics to which the NAMCP library does not have access, or that would be a duplication of efforts, thereby giving NAMCP members access to other databases and libraries while affording the same to other association members.

CONCLUSION

Doctors must become advocates for total quality care, which involves a coordinated effort on the part of providers and patients to improve the health status of the American public. Total quality care encompasses accessible health care and effective public and corporate policy in all aspects of the delivery system, including managed care organizations. For such an idea to work, though, physicians must proactively participate in the coordination of all aspects and parties in the health care delivery system. These include patients; academia; associations; employers; government; health insurance companies; hospitals; managed health care organizations; pharmaceuticals; and technology. Part of the process is to work toward changing the negative attitudes of practitioners and the public toward managed health care. The patient's initial interpretation of managed care defines it as a cost-cutting device for employers and the government. Many physicians have looked on managed care as a means of restricting physicians' incomes, controlling and second-guessing medical decisions, and adding various forms of regulation to their practices.

But these views are nonproductive. Physicians need to view managed health care as a potential solution to today's health care crisis. It is important for physicians to realize that by assuming a leadership role in the development and administration of managed health care, they can be instrumental in delivering care in a cost-effective manner, while maintaining the freedom to practice high-quality medicine. As managed health care progresses into the next century, physicians can be instrumental in heightening public awareness of the system's usefulness in controlling costs while delivering appropriate medical services.

The philosophy underlying the formation of the NAMCP is perhaps best summarized by Dr. William Glazer:

> It is obvious that managed care is here to stay. As idealistic as this may sound, it would be to the distinct advantage of every doctor in this country not only to adopt more positive attitudes and behaviors but also to learn to harness and use the potential benefits of managed care to optimal professional advantage. Managed care can be made to work for, not against, the physician.[5]

The managed health care industry has and will continue to change a great deal. Contrary to what many physicians think, the profession can maintain its life-style and status in a managed health care system comprised in whole or part of managed care, but adaptation and proactive participation in the future development of the system is vitally important for continued personal and professional growth.

NAMCP's definition of managed care is "managing the health care expenditure dollar while maintaining total quality care." The NAMCP was formed as an inclusive and constructive organization whose aims were to positively influence the health care industry and service the individual and collective needs of its physician members. As such, it welcomes the support and participation of all key constituencies, including health maintenance organizations and preferred provider executives; allied health professionals; medical schools; academicians; researchers; medical students and residents; government officials; pharmaceutical representatives; employers and human resource executives; the health insurance industry; and hospital management and administrators. Through this broad collaboration of influences, NAMCP hopes to both validate and prioritize physician concerns in dealing with managed health care matters into the next century.

The NAMCP strives to positively influence the managed health care environment by helping solve cost and financing problems as they arise. The association supports practicing physicians' interests and helps them survive and flourish in the managed health care arena by providing for their educational, research, and communication needs. By supporting physicians in this manner, the NAMCP promotes an environment that enables the managed health care system to maintain its focus of providing quality health care at a reasonable investment on the part of the government, employers, and patients.

The 1990s will be an interesting, experimental time for managed health care. Those on the cutting edge are constantly devising new combinations of prospective payment; case management; capitation; risk sharing; service and benefits mix; incentives; and prices. What is in existence today should by no means be counted as final. The entire managed care concept is still evolving.

In tomorrow's managed care system, the buyers will manage the care in addition to the costs. Major players in this system, including employers, unions, insurance companies, and the government, want to become more directly involved in financing and service delivery. Managed health care plans will find new methods of contracting with cooperating providers and in so doing, will forge a new and different relationship between health care purchasers and health care suppliers.

The challenge of managed care is here and now. For physicians and hospitals who believe that managed care will dominate the health care system of the 1990s, there are many opportunities to participate in the managed care movement. Just as managed care continues its growth in the managed health care arena, so, too, will the NAMCP. The association exists to serve and help physicians who work in managed health care of any form. It seeks to be open and positive in its mission and to encourage the professional growth of all those involved in the managed health care industry.

REFERENCES

1. White K. The era of teamwork: managed care comes of age. *Managed Care: A Guide for Physicians.* Spring 1992; 24.

2. Health Insurance Association of America. *The Fundamentals of Managed Care: Its History, Current Status, and Future.* Washington, DC: HIAA;October 1991:1–19.

3. Edwards JC, Donati RM. *Current Medical Practice: A Handbook for Residents and Medical Students.* St. Louis, MO: Group Health Foundation;1993:60–62.

4. The Society of Teachers of Family Medicine. *Managed Health Care: A Teaching Syllabus.* Kansas City, MO: Task Force on Managed Health Care. May 1990:6–7,18–23.

5. Glazer W. Doctor's response to managed care. *Medical Interface.* April 1992:14.

SUGGESTED READING

Coile RC Jr. *The New Medicine: Reshaping Medical Practice and Health Care Management,* Gaithersburg, MD: Aspen Publishers, Inc.;1990:133–145.

Preferred Provider Organizations: Productive Partnerships for Cost-Effective, Quality Health Care. American Association of Preferred Provider Organizations, 1988.

Editorial Commentary

Susan L. Howell
David B. Nash

Today, nearly half of all practicing physicians are involved in some form of managed health care delivery. Yet until recently, virtually no professional organization existed to serve the practicing managed care physician (as opposed to groups representing the interests of managed care plans, or physician managers). In 1991, the NAMCP was founded as a nonprofit, 501(c)6 association to serve as a resource on a national scale not only for managed care physicians, but all physicians who want to learn about managed care.

William C. Williams III, MD, a managed health care physician in family practice, is president and founder of the NAMCP. Dr. Williams has played an instrumental role in developing the "physicians' track" at the now annual National Managed Health Care Congress, a pivotal managed care forum held in Washington, D.C. each April. Dr. Williams has garnered the additional expertise of Daniel H. Friend, MBA, and R. S. Venable, MD, for this chapter. Both Mr. Friend and Dr. Venable were among the key players who helped realize Dr. Williams's vision of a professional association managed "by and for" practicing physicians. Mr. Friend is executive vice president and director of programs and services for the NAMCP, and Dr. Venable, who is chief medical officer for Humana Health Plan in Tampa Bay, Florida is a member of the NAMCP's advisory board and editor of the NAMCP professional journal.

The authors have described for us the history of the NAMCP's creation, including an overview of the role of managed care in today's health care delivery system and the historical paucity of information and representative organizations for physicians interested in managed care. They have also provided a comprehensive look at NAMCP's mission; the many ways in which physicians (and medical students) can become involved; and its plans for the future. The authors emphasize that the NAMCP is, above all, a resource, a means for physicians to become proactive participants within the managed health care arena. As a nonpolitical entity, it is distinguishable from, for example, a labor union; its purpose is not, the authors maintain, to effect change per se, but rather to advocate for the practicing managed care physician through education, research, and communication.

Although in its infancy, the NAMCP has achieved an impressive array of objectives. Since its inception in 1991, its membership has virtually exploded to 12,000 at the time of this writing. Though MDs and DOs comprise the majority of NAMCP members, managed care executives and businesses affiliated with managed care are represented as well. NAMCP members receive its quarterly newsletter and (soon to be published) academic journal, which will offer comprehensive coverage of clinical practice and management issues.

The NAMCP cannot be accused of maintaining a low profile. Among the highlights of the organization's 1993 schedule:

- sponsorship of a regional forum on health care reform in Tampa, Florida
- sponsorship of a national symposium focusing on physician-hospital organization (PHO) development in Orlando, Florida
- cosponsorship of the Third National Managed Care Forum, sponsored by the American Hospital Association's Society for Health Care Planning and Marketing
- cosponsorship of the Individual Case Management Association's annual conference
- cosponsorship of the regional and national meetings of the National Managed Health Care Congress.

In addition to fostering interprofessional and physician-patient relationships through participation in regional and national conferences, the NAMCP is committed to the ongoing professional development of its members through efforts such as a monograph series on legal contracting issues, which it sponsors with the National Health Lawyers Association, and a series on communication.

Particularly exciting was the launching of two formal educational programs, the Managed Care Medical Director's Institute for

Managed Care, a five-day program through Northwestern University, scheduled for Spring 1994; and the School for Managed Care, a two-day program to be held in various sites around the country, beginning in late 1993/early 1994. CME credit will be available for both programs. These programs are the first to offer continuing education to physicians that is solely managed care-oriented. The NAMCP is also working toward collaborative relationships with medical schools to develop a managed health care curriculum. Eventually, the authors would like to see the NAMCP become the credentialing body for managed care physicians. Other planned events for 1994 include sponsorship of the Clinical Outcomes/Research Conference, to be held in New Orleans; and the NAMCP National Conference, to be held in Phoenix.

With its dizzying array of involvements and substantial long-term goals, the NAMCP promises to be a growing presence within the medical profession and the health care industry. There is much work to be done, and the NAMCP is one group demonstrating its willingness and capacity to carry out this agenda, further evidenced by its meeting with the Clinton administration's task force on health care reform. In the NAMCP, managed care physicians can find a long-awaited common voice.

Chapter 6

Toward Cost-Effective Health Care

David J. Shulkin
Alan H. Rosenstein

As health care dollars become an increasingly limited resource, more efficient utilization of health care services has become an imperative. The federal government has turned to managed care and other cost containment strategies as a primary vehicle for reducing our national health care debt. Despite their emphasis on cost restrictions, health maintenance organizations (HMOs) have been found to provide quality of care as good or better than that of the fee-for-service setting.[1-5] Physicians in managed care organizations provide a lower intensity of care than fee-for-service physicians without a documented worsening of outcomes.[6-9] In addition, HMO physicians are less likely to hospitalize patients and perform unnecessary surgeries.[10,11] Over 90 percent of health maintenance organizations use physicians as gatekeepers to decide what services will be necessary for their patients.[12]

Most practicing physicians, however, have few places to turn for learning how to practice in a cost-effective manner. Academic medical institutions too often focus on the care of the critically ill and patients with rare diagnoses. Students are taught to "leave no stone unturned" in their diagnostic journeys and to rely upon the most sophisticated technologies. Managed care organizations have in large part kept their distance from the large teaching centers because of their lack of enthusiasm for subsidizing educational costs. As a result, few physicians in training are exposed to managed care philosophies and the case management approach to patient care.

The gap between what is taught and what is expected of physicians in today's changing health care arena is becoming increasingly apparent as more physicians enter managed care organizations directly from residency programs. This chapter was prepared with both the practicing physician and the physician-manager in mind. We will present both the background and principles necessary to understand the theory of cost-effective care as well as specific applications of this developing aspect of patient care.

FORCES DRIVING HEALTH CARE COSTS

At the end of 1992, U.S. expenditures for health care services amounted to almost $800 billion, accounting for more than 12 percent of the gross national product.[13] Some experts predict that health care spending will climb to the trillion dollar mark by the year 2000. This is nearly 15 percent of the gross national product and almost double the spending for health care services in Canada and other European countries. The various sectors have tried in their respective ways to reduce their financial health care burdens. A priority of the federal government (the largest purchaser of health care services, at 42 percent) is its continued ability to support the Medicare and Medicaid programs. Private industry, the second-largest purchaser of health care services (37 percent), is concerned about the 25 percent in annual corporate profits consumed by health care costs. Individual consumers compose the third-largest purchaser of health care services; they are concerned about quality, cost, and continuous coverage.

Before we begin our efforts to cure the system, we must first examine the forces responsible for the current health care crisis.

Health Care Access/Third-Party Payers

Providing health care for the estimated 37 million Americans who are uninsured is arguably one reason our health care costs are so high. In addition, the majority of those covered by health insurance are covered by some type of indemnity, third-party health care insurance provided through their employers. Employers' subsidization of health insurance costs has the effect of insulating individuals from the "real" costs of health care, and serves as a disincentive to investigate cost-effective alternatives.

Fee-for-Service, Supply-Driven System

In the traditional fee-for-services insurance system, providers are paid for services rendered. This has the effect of creating a supply-driven system in which there is no economic incentive to be cost-conscious about health care delivery. It is important to note that fee-for-service does not directly increase supply, but it does little to encourage cost-efficiency.

Health Care Technology/Labor and Supplies

The direct costs of purchasing the latest in health care technology add significantly to our health care debt. We also have to pass on the cost of labor and supplies needed to support this technology. Physicians are taught to embrace the "latest and greatest" in technological advancements, with scant awareness of the cost of providing such services.

Patient Demand/Customary Care

Americans are accustomed to treatment on demand.[14] Patients are accustomed to receiving all the services requested in a timely fashion, but are the treatments they request always appropriate? Can we afford to continue to provide an unlimited number of services to an unlimited number of people without regard to potential for recovery or quality of life? One in every seven health care dollars is purportedly devoted to treatment given during the last several days of life.[15] Arriving at a solution to our nation's health care woes requires us to examine these and other hard questions not only in monetary terms, but in a moral and ethical light.

System Waste/Inefficiency

Many authorities suggest that 20 to 40 percent of the health care provided does not contribute to improvements in patient care.[16] One can point to the waste and inefficiencies incurred by bureaucratic management. A recent article in the *New England Journal of Medicine* estimated that 19 to 24 percent of the national health care dollar is being spent solely on administrative costs incurred from monitoring the health care system.[17] Another culprit is equivocal or clinically unjustified treatments and procedures. Several articles appearing in the *Journal of the American Medical Association*, the *New England Journal of Medicine*, and other reputable medical journals have suggested that a significant percentage of treatments, surgeries, and procedures may not be clinically justified,[18-21] including coronary angiography, coronary artery bypass surgery, carotid endarterectomy, Caesarean sections, hysterectomies, and endoscopies. (See Figure 6–1.)

Physician Demand: Offensive/Defensive

Are most physicians aware of the costs of the services they are ordering? Many studies suggest they are not.[22-25] From the moment

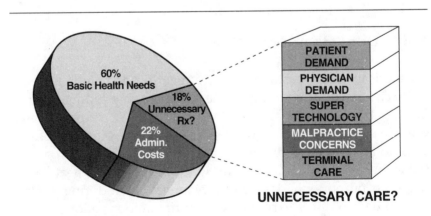

Figure 6–1 Health Cost Distribution

we enter medical school and throughout our residency and fellowship training, we are encouraged to use all the resources at our disposal to provide effective and comprehensive diagnosis and treatment. We are taught to equate quality with quantity. Kassirer and Johnson have referred to this phenomenon as "our stubborn quest for diagnostic certainty."[26,27] This is an example of "offensive" physician behavior responsible for driving up health care costs. Practicing defensively has come to characterize the way we practice medicine in this country. Even the most cost-conscious physician has been motivated to perform additional tests for fear of malpractice reprisal.

REACTION BY THE FEDERAL GOVERNMENT AND PRIVATE SECTOR

The government is blessed with the power of legislation. Its most ambitious attempt to control health care spending occurred with the 1982 Tax Equity and Fiscal Responsibility Act (TEFRA) legislation, which had a dramatic effect on hospital-related care for two important reasons. First, it paved the way for utilization review by establishing statewide peer review organizations (PROs) to monitor the appropriateness and quality of care for all Medicare hospital admissions. By establishing standard severity of illness and intensity of service criteria, hospitals were to be paid only if the services provided were deemed clinically appropriate at the hospital (acute) level of care. For the first time, the concept of financial risk was introduced in regard to potential payment denials for nonapproved care. Second, it paved the way for direct reimbursement limitations by switching inpatient care payments from fee-for-service to a case-based diagnosis-related group (DRG) reimbursement system. The second component of financial risk was thus introduced. With a fixed-case lump sum reimbursement, financial incentives became directly linked to efficiency and expediency of care. On the heels of the government's initiatives, the private sector was free to flex its muscle in the marketplace. Discounted contractual care quickly became the competitive norm, spawning the birth of managed care as we know it today.

What have been the results of these programs? On the cost-savings side, hospital admissions, patient days, and lengths of stay have decreased dramatically, with obvious reductions for inpatient spending, although some might argue that the dollars saved from the reduction in inpatient services have merely been passed on to the outpatient sector. Despite the cutbacks in inpatient care, quality of care seems to have improved. This is probably a result of holding providers more directly accountable for services rendered, which obliges them to pay more attention to the appropriateness and process of health care delivery.[28] Recent government incentives for cost control have extended the concept of per-case reimbursement to include outpatient services, lumping hospital and physician payments on a per-case basis for certain procedures (e.g., coronary artery bypass graft [CABG]), and revising the outpatient fee schedule for physician payments.

HEALTH CARE COST CONTROL: STRATEGIES AND INCENTIVES

Has managed care been successful in controlling health care costs? A recent article in the *Wall Street Journal* summarized the differences in 1991 average annual employee premiums based on insurance category. A typical indemnity premium averaged $3,573, while a typical PPO averaged $3,355, and a typical HMO averaged $3,046 per employee.[29] These cost savings are possible because of the interaction of several different forces. First, physicians involved in HMO networks are indoctrinated into a system that stresses efficiency of care. Second, managed care organizations employ many strategies to assist their physician staff with strategies to lower the cost of care. The most direct way to encourage change in behavior and performance is to link change with economic incentives. Economic incentives for physicians and hospitals are presented in Table 6–1. Aligning physicians' rewards with those of the manged care organization is usually quite effective. This often works best when physicians are staff members of

Table 6–1 Economic Incentives by Payer Mix

Economic Incentive	Admission	Length of Stay	Resources Used
For Hospitals			
Full charge*	+	+	+
Discounted charges†	+?	+?	+?
Payment per case‡	+?	–	–
Payment per diem§	+?	+??	–
Capitation‖	–	–	–
For Physicians			
Full charge*	+	+	+
Discounted charges¶	+	+	+
Payment per case#	+?	+	+
Payment per diem**	+	+?	+?
Capitation‖††	–	–	–

+ = desireable/increase, – = undesireable/decrease

*Reimbursed for services provided. For physicians, fee–for–service.
†PPOs: Reimbursed on percentage of charges; the question is whether discounted reimbursement is enough to cover costs.
‡Prospective payment (DRGs): Fixed payment, with the emphasis to do less; the question is that it is subject to "admission approval."
§Medicaid: Paid by the day, with the emphasis to do less; the questions are that it is subject to "admission approval" and payment may be only for "medically necessary" days.
‖Payment per enrollee (HMOs): Money is paid "up front," with incentive to do less.
¶PPOs: Same incentives as for fee–for–service.
#Medicare (DRGs): Physicians are reimbursed for services provided; the question is that Medicare may deny payment for unnecessary services.
**Medicaid: Physicians are reimbursed for services provided; the question is that Medicaid may deny payment for unnecessary services.
††Physicians may be on fee–for–service reimbursement with hospital on capitation.

Source: Reprinted from *The Western Journal of Medicine,* Vol. 154, No. 2, p. 177, with permission of the California Medical Association, © 1991.

the corporation (i.e., have a vested financial interest)—as is the case in the traditional closed-panel HMO—as opposed to a network model, where a comparatively small percentage of HMO patients may be treated. Other cost-restrictive mechanisms include selective credentialing and more aggressive utilization controls, such as utilization review.

The potential downside of influencing behavior by incentives is that the focus remains solely on the cost of care, and little emphasis is likely to be placed on the quality or appropriateness of the care delivered. Some organizations have begun to reward financially for an assessment of quality. Most notable among these organizations is U.S. Healthcare, an independent practice association (IPA) in Blue Bell, Pennsylvania. Skeptics to this approach are taking a "wait and see" attitude because of their belief that quality care is inherently difficult to quantify.

Physician Education: The Key to Promoting Cost-Effective Care

We have briefly discussed some of the most common strategies for inhibiting health care costs, including administrative interventions, financial incentives, and monitoring of medical care decisions. Common to all is the recognition that physicians control an estimated 80 percent of all health care costs.[30] Programs that do not achieve physician acceptance have been shown time and time again to fail. It has been found that physicians prefer an educational approach to cost issues,[31] and that efforts aimed at educating physicians about the cost of care and other cost-containment techniques can significantly lower the cost of care.[24] Education must therefore remain the central effort in promoting cost-effective changes in practice behavior.

Physician participation in cost containment efforts has not been easy. The basic instincts and philosophies that guide the physician have their origins in medical school and academic training. A physician may say, "I've been in practice for 20 years now and I don't see why I have to change." Traditionally, physicians have been relatively autonomous—and function as creatures of habit. This makes it difficult to motivate physicians to change. Some are more resistant than others. Older physicians approaching retirement age, for example, are predictably less open to change. The young physician is more familiar with the changing environment of health care delivery and is therefore less entrenched in traditionalism and more apt to be flexible.

Educational initiatives can be conducted at several levels. First, education in the tenets of cost-effective, quality care must begin in medical school. Also, more opportunities are needed for applied learning throughout training.

Good medical care will never be cheap. However, there is much doctors can do to lower costs. Established physicians can help by sharing their cost-effective expertise with younger physicians. Forums for information exchange, such as educational seminars, can familiarize physicians with the economic realities impacting their practices. For example, whether seasoned or new, all physicians can benefit from gleaning the fallacy in the "quantity equals quality" imperative. Likewise, physicians can also be encouraged to learn the costs of the tests they order. In a survey of medical students, resident physicians, and faculty, each underestimated the charge for common tests by a factor of nearly three.[25] However, an inverse relationship has been found between number of tests ordered and the level of physician training.[32, 33] In general, it is fair to say that few physicians have knowledge of the prices of even the most common tests they order. When doctors are aware of the costs of tests, there is a 31 percent decrease in testing volume.[34] Physicians have to ask themselves if the test in question will positively impact patient management or improve quality of care.

By relying on the caveat "Do no harm," the more experienced physician can impart to those less experienced that while thorough evaluations are often reassuring to both patient and physician, exposing patients to unnecessary or duplicative testing or procedures may put them at greater risk for an adverse event. Some studies are invasive and can be associated with unnecessary morbidity, in addition to false positive results that can trigger a new series of tests and evaluations. In addition, excessive testing may yield only minimal incremental beneficial information. We call this the "rule of diminishing returns." Do what needs to be done in an efficient, judicious manner. Appropriate chart documentation stating your thoughts about the case is better protection than chasing results through additional testing.

In regard to concerns about malpractice, until tort reform finally has its day, physicians will unfortunately feel obliged to continue to order multiple tests and procedures in fear of potential retrospective malpractice claims. However, a better safeguard for the physician is to keep accurate, detailed medical record documentation. This includes a description of your thoughts on the case, why you are pursuing a particular clinical course, and your long-term follow-up plan.

Many physicians, primarily those in the hospital setting who provide care on a fee-for-service basis, remain unaware that additional testing does not equal additional reimbursement for the hospital. This is a good time for a crash course in the newly implemented revised reimbursement schedules. Increasingly, pre-determined fee scales and utilization review are being integrated into the fee-for-service reimbursement system.

Physicians frequently argue that charge information bears little resemblance to cost information and therefore has little relevance. Charges are still based on some degree of cost and effort, and serve as a fair indicator of resource consumption. Hospitals with a cost accounting system can counter this issue more effectively by presenting actual cost data. While some hospitals still maintain a high charge schedule in order to gain additional revenues from that rare fee-for-service patient (in an effort to cost-shift dollars to cover the lower reimbursements offered by other payers), many are beginning to adjust their pricing structures to more accurately reflect the actual cost of services provided.

Practice Guidelines

The recognition that unnecessary services contribute to rising medical costs has helped push the development of practice guidelines. Numerous professional organizations, government agencies, and health care providers have begun to produce these guidelines for a variety of clinical conditions. One method of guideline development is to form standards of practice by initiating a literature review of the subject, reviewing the data, and then developing a group consensus on the guideline content. Anecdotal evidence suggests that guidelines may be best accepted, and compliance is therefore best, when physicians or opinion leaders in their institution have been actively involved in their development.[35] Studies that examined the impact of guidelines on cost have demonstrated that substantial reductions in resource use occurred, with no demonstrable adverse affect on quality of care.[36]

Information Sharing

An alternate approach to improving quality and lowering cost, while stimulating change in physician behavior, is information sharing. Physicians tend to practice in an "information void." While there is comfort in adhering to standards established by our colleagues, we really do not know much about the performance of the group as a whole.[37] Information sharing allows, through profiling, the comparison with peers of physician practice patterns. The goal of information sharing is to examine variations in care through physician education and feedback in order to further the development of guidelines, critical pathways, and recommended treatment protocols. In this way, physicians are encouraged to participate in the process of continuous quality improvement. Information sharing also offers the opportunity for physicians and hospitals to work together toward improving the process of care.[38] The other reality is that payers, who contract with providers who can demonstrate more efficient performance profiles,[39, 40] are increasingly requiring managed care organizations and hospitals to provide performance and cost data.

While we firmly believe in the importance of information exchange, it is critical that this information be presented in a constructive manner. Information sharing runs the danger of being construed as a means of isolating the "bad apples" or "economic credentialing." We also feel that internally driven data systems are preferable to externally driven profiles, the latter offering little or no opportunity for physician input.

Much can be gained by information sharing among different disciplines of physicians on the topic of cost. One organization, Physicians for Research in Cost-Effectiveness (PRICE), has initiated a forum for physicians to share ideas about cost-effective care. PRICE publishes a newsletter (available through the American College of Physician Executives in Tampa, Florida) that details information about cost-effective practice innovations. For example, PRICE conducted a survey that revealed that 75 percent of nephrologists do not do a metabolic workup on a patient with his or her first kidney stone[31] and few ear, nose, and throat (ENT) specialists order routine X-rays in the diagnosis of sinusitis. Although these results are not based upon scientific sampling techniques, they do provide a basis for discussion among physicians on ways to promote cost-effective practice behavior. Several surgeons who were PRICE members shared their findings that internists order too many tests before referring patients. (Many internists believe they are simply providing a more detailed evaluation for the surgeon, although in fact it may be better to discuss with the surgeon which tests are truly necessary.)

One group in particular that has much to gain from enhanced communication is surgeons and pathologists. One pathologist noted 41 different specimens from anal tags to vascular graft thrombi that are routinely submitted to his department; his recommendation was that referrals are inappropriate if they look grossly normal and are uncomplicated. Other physicians have suggested that nursing home patients do well with a drug holiday one day per week, cutting drug costs by one-seventh. One California physician reported that his hospital saved more than $100,000 a year by detecting fecal impaction before performing a barium enema. Another hospital saved $40,000 a year by eliminating disposable hand brushes and employing reusables in the operating room. Alone, these ideas will do little to impact health care costs. Their utility is as good as the momentum generated through physician collaboration and communication.

In regard to physicians' reliance on cutting-edge technology and the ensuing impact on health care costs, one study has shown that physicians are adept at embracing the latest technology but they still continue to utilize the older, more conventional modalities.[41] Cost considerations aside, however, residents have become so entrenched in using technology to make a diagnosis that the routine history and physical—the major foci in making an accurate diagnosis—are often underemphasized or overlooked. The technologic imperative, in the authors' opinion, can act as a barrier to more interactive patient-physician communication. We advocate the use of the latest technology if the diagnostic yield is optimal.

Finally, for those employed in the hospital sector, a word about hospital loyalty, economic survival, and the philosophical imperative of allocating care. It used to be that if one was dissatisfied working at a particular hospital, one could simply move to the hospital across the street. Today, all hospitals are likely to be suffering from the same economic constraints as the one with whom we are presently employed. We must be prepared for any number of changes in our workplaces, whether in referral patterns, restricted privileges, or radical alteration of customary amenities, from operating room schedules to physician lounge conveniences.

The goals of managed care cannot be realized without the active consent and involvement of physicians. Physicians, patients, and providers stand to be rewarded by a system built on a foundation of cost-efficiency and continuous quality improvement: payers will benefit from a better value for their money; patients will benefit from more appropriate allocation and access to health care resources; and physicians will benefit from happier, healthier patients.

BASIC CONCEPTS OF COST-EFFECTIVENESS

In today's environment, few people would argue that there is an unlimited amount of resources to devote to health care. The methods of cost-effectiveness analysis provide one mechanism for making rational decisions about where to direct resources. Cost-effectiveness models can help answer questions such as "What is my confidence level if I am only 95 percent sure I have the right diagnosis?" Similarly, if $500 is spent and a diagnostic confidence level of 95 percent is reached, should an additional $500 be spent to increase our confidence level to 96 percent?

The individual physician will most likely interact with data on cost-effectiveness from readings in the literature, reports at conferences or meetings, and from on-site studies based on large patient population analyses. Rarely will he or she do a cost-effectiveness analysis to decide how to care for his or her patients. Many would argue that even if there was a means to perform such a complex calculation, it would be inappropriate to do so. The donning of the role of resource allocator is not comfortable for the vast majority of physicians. Even so, the average physician, on a daily basis, makes hundreds of informal cost-effectiveness decisions, such as whether the extra money spent for a test or drug jusitifies the anticipated clinical outcome.[42]

Economic Analysis Studies

In the area of economic analyses, there are three common types of studies performed: (1) cost-identification, (2) cost-effectiveness, and (3) cost-benefit. Cost-identification studies help determine the cost of a particular course of treatment. These studies usually serve to identify the least costly method of treatment. For example, is it less costly to treat a patient with gallstones with a laparoscopic cholecystectomy or a traditional laparotomy? Cost identification studies should be used to guide clinical decisions only if the intervention is less expensive *and* has an outcome better than or at least equal to the alternative.

Cost-effectiveness studies are most useful in comparing one type of medical intervention to another and should not be considered in isolation from other treatment options. In evaluating the cost-effectiveness of a particular product or a diagnostic or therapeutic intervention, the concepts of efficacy, effectiveness, and efficiency must be addressed. Simply put, efficacy is whether the product or intervention works under ideal circumstances; effectiveness is whether that product or intervention works under real world conditions; and efficiency is whether the best outcome is obtained for the money spent.[42]

Cost-effectiveness studies also address an outcomes component. Results of these studies are usually expressed in the cost per unit of improved outcome.[42] For example, the results of this analysis could be expressed in dollars per year of life saved. A more sophisticated way of expressing outcomes is the quality adjusted life years (QUALYs) saved. The idea behind the QUALY is that not all life years saved are of equal value.[42] In other words, a year of life spent in a coma attached to a ventilator is not equal to a year of a fully productive life. The QUALY is fast becoming the preferred method of expressing results in cost-effectiveness studies.

When comparing cost-effective analysis results to decide how much more expensive one strategy is than another, most effective strategy, cost-effective ratios (costs divided by the effectiveness of the intervention) can be misleading. For example, if one drug is much more expensive than another but produces a slightly better outcome, is it worth it? In this case, incremental cost-effectiveness ratios may be more useful. This ratio is the cost of the new strategy over the old, divided by the difference in effectiveness.[43] Analysis of additional cost and additional clinical outcomes of alternative interventions is called *incremental analysis.*[42]

The third type of study commonly seen is the cost-benefit analysis. In this study both costs and outcomes are reported in dollars. If the benefits outweigh the costs, the intervention in question is likely to be a useful clinical strategy. The greatest difficulty in cost-benefit analyses is that it can be extremely difficult to translate an outcome—such as the ability to live one year longer—into a monetary value.

When evaluating economic analysis, it is essential to understand the point of view from which the study was conducted. There are generally four recognized points of views: (1) society's, (2) the patient's, (3) the payer's, and (4) the provider's.[42] The point of view from which the study was undertaken may have a dramatic impact on interpretation. For example, lowering the length of an inpatient hospital stay may substantially reduce the cost of care to the hospital (the provider), but if the patient is unable to care for him or herself, the cost to the patient and his or her family (who may need to stay home to care for the patient) is likely to increase; and medical supplies may need to be purchased.

Another important facet of economic evaluations concerns studies that evaluate the appropriateness of care. Several studies stand out as having had a large impact on shaping the direction of health policy. The first of this type of research can be traced back to John Wennberg, a professor of medicine at Dartmouth Medical School in Hanover, New Hampshire. In the 1970s, Dr. Wennberg documented large variations in the type of care delivered to residents of various New England towns. Some of the variations were tremendous. For example, age-adjusted rates for surgical procedures such as hysterectomies, prostatectomies, and tonsillectomies varied several fold among different parts of a state.[44] The implication of the Wennberg study was that if doctors practice medicine differently, some portion of their practices is resulting in the delivery of unnecessary or inefficient care. The first major study to address this issue was published in 1984 when researchers from the RAND Corporation in Santa Monica, California, examined the appropriateness of four major surgical procedures. The results suggested that possibly as many as 64 percent of carotid endarterectomies, as well as procedures such as coronary artery bypass surgeries, were being done for inappropriate reasons.[45] This report received a great deal of attention and contributed to the rapid increase in medical care monitoring that continues today.

Economic studies have become more frequent in the medical literature. For example, one report concluded that 30 to 59 percent of the 4 million stool studies for culture of ova and parasites are unwarranted. By simply limiting these studies to patients who have been hospitalzed for four days or less, the vast majority of unnecessary tests can be eliminated.[46] Another report found that 70 percent of routine coagulation studies can be avoided by following physician-developed guidelines.[43] This would amount to a savings of $61,000 per year in the authors' hospital alone. Pharyngeal cultures for gonorrhea in adolescent girls add a cost of more than $11,000 for each additional case found.[47] (Selective use of pharyngeal cultures is advocated.) Deyo and his colleagues found, in a selected cohort of patients with back pain, that education can replace lumbar spine X-rays without impacting the satisfaction of care.[48]

Given the fact that economic research in health care is in its infancy, it cannot provide all the answers about cost-effective approaches to patient care. In fact, the majority of physicians' clinical decisions are based on past experience and sometimes gut instinct. As previously discussed, guidance for decisions about efficient approaches to patient care can sometimes best be obtained by learning what our colleagues are doing.

Specific Areas of Cost-Effective Interventions

We next review a cost-effective study using some specific instances of diagnostic testing as examples of cost-effective practice.

Efficient Practices in Utilizing Routine Labs

Biochemical screening has become routine. Automated machines run panels of blood chemistries for the price of a single test. Yet, these prices may be deceiving. The greater the number of tests run from a single specimen, the greater the chance that a result will fall outside the normal range.[49] If a panel is run with 20 tests, there is only a 36 percent chance that all the results will be normal.[50] Results that fall outside the normal range are often false positive tests. In the case of an asymptomatic patient, the physician is faced with the dilemma of ignoring the result, repeating the test, or doing a further diagnostic evaluation. The latter two options may add further unnecessary costs to the patient's care, yet in today's environment of chart reviews for quality of care and monitoring by peer review organizations, it is hard to ignore abnormal test results.

Again, before ordering a test, it is necessary to weigh the potential benefit to the patient against the cost of the test. Physicians must also consider the cost of follow-up tests when abnormal results are apparent. One strategy that can help avoid this dilemma is to simply not order tests that are likely to have a low positive predictive value. The positive predictive value defines the probability of a disease being present if a test result is positive. It is calculated from the sensitivity, specificity, and prevalence of disease, and the presence of test abnormality.[51]

Laboratory tests with a low predictive value may fall outside the normal range and add little to the clinical evaluation of the patient. For example, serum chloride is run routinely on electrolyte panels, yet it provides little useful information in the routine setting. Elevated chloride values are nonspecific, as are decreased chloride values. Chloride values are useful in the calculation of the anion gap in the setting of a metabolic acidosis and in severe electrolyte disorders. However, the positive predictive value of serum chloride in the routine patient population is low and an abnormal chloride is unlikely to play an important diagnostic role in the care of most patients.

Measurements of serum carbon dioxide, lactic dehydrogenase, erythrocyte sedimentation rates, and urinary urobilinogen also may not be cost-effective, especially as routine screening tests, because of their low predictive value in patients without clinical abnormalities.[49] Other tests—low blood urea nitrogen value, abnormal mean corpuscular hemoglobin, elevated uric acid, or abnormal urinary sediment—given to asymptomatic patients are often not worth pursuing with further diagnostic studies. If abnormal results have no correlation with clinical findings, the physician should refrain from pursuing workups for the purpose of satisfying curiosity or obtaining diagnostic certainty.[52]

A laboratory result outside the reference range does not necessarily mean that there is something wrong with the patient. Technical errors can contribute to inaccurate results, as can sampling techniques, diet, activity, and medications. In addition, normal values are often not adjusted for age or sex.[53] When a physician chooses not to repeat or pursue abnormal laboratory results, proper documentation of a reasonable thought process will satisfy peer review groups that monitor medical decisions. It is hard to argue with sound medical judgment.

Preoperative Labs

Few topics have received closer scrutiny than the preoperative evaluation. Yet, routine preoperative screening remains commonplace. What follows is a review of the literature and recommendations meant to generate meaningful discussions among clinicians interested in developing policies for preoperative labs within their organizations.

The Preoperative Chest X-Ray. The purpose of a preoperative chest X-ray is to identify conditions that could influence operative or postoperative conditions. These include findings such as tracheal deviation, mediastinal masses, or cardiomegaly. Studies have shown that these abnormalities increase with age. A retrospective study of 797 preoperative chest X-rays revealed abnormalities in 17 percent of persons over age 60, and only 2 percent in those under 60.[54] Another study showed that of 1,000 patients who had preoperative chest X-rays, abnormalities were much more frequent (30 percent) in patients over age 50 than in younger patients (3 percent).[55] Though age is often used as a guideline for ordering preoperative chest X-rays, there are no established standards dictating who should receive one. The Mayo Clinic requires chest X-rays for patients 60 and older, those with histories of cardiac or pulmonary disease, or those with recent respiratory symptoms.[56] The American College of Physicians suggests that advancing age should not be the sole indication for a preoperative X-ray,[57] as the presence of abnormalities does not necessarily justify their examination.

The alternative to using age as a strict criteria is using greater reliance on clinical judgment. In one study, a history and physical examination were found to identify a population of patients at low risk for having abnormal chest X-rays. Of 368 patients identified to have low-risk factors, only one was found to have an abnormal chest X-ray, and this did not affect the surgery.[58] In patients with chest X-ray abnormalities but normal history and physical examinations, outcomes are rarely affected. Of the six patients with X-ray abnormalities without symptoms or suggestive history, none had a change in clinical outcome because of X-ray findings. Often chest X-rays are ordered for use as a baseline study in postoperative care. A study completed by the American College of Physicians could not demonstrate the need for a baseline preoperative chest X-ray when a patient had a postop chest complication.[59]

Complete Blood Cell Counts (CBC). There is little evaluation of the preoperative CBC. The Mayo Clinic does not require a CBC on a patient under 60 unless that patient is having a Type & Screen or a Type & Cross.[56] Other institutions have initiated policies for preoperative CBCs in all female patients; male patients over age 40, surgical procedures with anticipated significant blood loss, malignancies, anticoagulant use, renal disease, or smokers with a greater than 20-pack year history.

Chemistries. Routine preoperative laboratory screening among 3,782 low-risk patients revealed only one abnormality that resulted in an initiation of a new treatment.[56] Robins and Mushlin found that screening with BUN/CR would detect an estimated three cases of renal insufficiency among 10,000 surgical patients in whom this disorder was known to previously exist.[60] Aspartate aminotransferase measurement would detect 2.5 cases of occult hepatitis per 10,000 patients, and a two-hour postprandial glucose would detect 29 per 10,000 cases of diabetes. The American College of Physicians' handbook suggests that biochemical profiles are not routinely indicated for preoperative testing.[57] The Mayo Clinic requires only creatinine and glucose testing in patients over 40.[56] In addition, patients who are taking diuretics or undergoing bowel preparation have a potassium measurement.

Use of Prior Lab Tests

A study of 7,549 preoperative tests indicated that 47 percent were repeats of tests performed in the previous year. Of those tests defined as normal, 0.4 percent of repeat serologic values prior to surgery were outside a range considered acceptable for surgery.[61] In the majority of serologic values that were abnormal after being repeated, a chart review indicated that there had been a clinical change. Of those patients with abnormal lab values, the repeat testing confirmed the abnormality in 17 percent of the patients. The authors recommend that tests (CBC, electrolytes, prothrombin time/partial thromboplastin time [PT/PTT]) be used within four months of preoperative evaluation. Clinicians who feel uncomfortable about not screening preoperatively could use the results of previous tests. If the previous tests are normal and there has been no change in the patient's clinical state, repeat testing is not necessary. Patients having electrolyte surgery could be safely tested preoperatively—if indicated—up to four months before the procedure. Data also suggest there is little reason to repeat an electrocardiogram (EKG) within a reasonable period if little change is expected. Rabkin and Horne examined the frequency of new abnormalities within two years of old EKGs. It was less than 10 percent in patients under 60 and 22 percent in patients over 60.[62]

COST-EFFICIENT CARE: MEDICAL RESOURCE MANAGEMENT

Medical resource management focuses on the efficiency and effectiveness of medical care. It is the third component contributing to a comprehensive system of high quality, cost-effective care (see Exhibit 6-1). The other two components are quality assessment and improvement. These components reduce unwanted events, and improve the process of care and the implementation of utilization management in order to ensure appropriate and expedient medical care.

The implementation of resource management as a tool for managing financial risk for services rendered is growing in popularity. The remainder of this section will focus on the Resource Management/Outcome Measurement Model we have developed at our hospital.

Medical resource management is a process involving five key steps. Exhibit 6–2 outlines the basic model of medical resource management. Step one of this process is to identify your priorities. What do you really want to study? Priorities can be identified by high volume, high cost or high risk admissions or procedures, or you may simply want to do special studies in an area that may benefit from more intensive study. Step two involves the method of data analysis. Data can be organized by hospital, department, diagnosis, ancillary service, or physician. Table 6–2 shows an example of how we evaluated the top 25 diagnoses in the hospital by volume and charges.

Steps three and four, involving data collection and dissemination, are the most crucial. Again, we cannot emphasize enough

---

Exhibit 6–1 High Quality Cost–Effective Care

I. Quality Assessment and Improvement
  – Reduce adverse outcomes
  – Reduce unwanted events
  – Reduce complications
  – Improve the process of care

II. Effective Utilization Management
  – Expedient treatment
  – Appropriate level of care
  – Length of stay—documentation

III. Efficient Resource Management
  – Reduce unnecessary services
  – Avoid duplication of services
  – Substitute less costly services
  – Emphasize cost-effective diagnosis and treatment
  – Encourage outpatient care

Exhibit 6–2 Medical Resource Management

I. Identify Priorities
  – High volume/high cost/high risk
  – Special studies
II. Data Analysis
  – By hospital/by department/by diagnosis
  – By ancillary service
  – By physician
III. Develop Alternatives
IV. Encourage Change
  – Information sharing
  – Physician participation
  – Medical staff leadership
V. Agents of Change
  – Protocols/guidelines
  – Critical pathways
  – Intensive utilization review
  – Computer–assisted suggestions
  – Physician education

Table 6–2 Top 25 Diagnoses by Volume

ICD-9 Code	Principal Diagnosis	Total Cases	LOS, Days	Gross Revenue	Net Revenue	Operating Costs	Profit/ Loss	Total Days
1 V3000	Single liveborn	2,810	3	9,435,825	5,647,153	5,322,889	324,264	10,381
2 V5810	Main. chemotherapy	252	2	1,319,006	874,040	769,043	104,996	689
3 65421	Prev. C-section	241	3	1,309,433	809,712	929,302	(119,590)	894
–	–	–	–	–	–	–	–	–
–	–	–	–	–	–	–	–	–
7 49391	Status asthmaticus	157	3	904,481	445,858	528,981	(83,123)	552
8 42800	Cong. heart failure	149	7	1,889,344	965,173	1,238,156	(272,982)	1,097
–	–	–	–	–	–	–	–	–
–	–	–	–	–	–	–	–	–
12 48600	Pneumonia org. nos	137	6	1,301,218	757,342	797,824	(40,482)	831
–	–	–	–	–	–	–	–	–
–	–	–	–	–	–	–	–	–
19 43600	Gastroenteritis	90	2	277,644	199,220	186,431	12,789	262
20 43600	CVA	85	6	699,078	495,639	458,873	36,766	577
21 78020	Syncope & collapse	83	3	440,519	250,409	299,774	(49,365)	256
–	–	–	–	–	–	–	–	–
24 78650	Chest pain nos	80	2	373,160	172,453	257,381	(84,928)	176

Source: Reprinted from Rosenstein, A., "Utilization review: Health economics and cost–effective management," in *Quality Assurance and Utilization Review,* Vol. 16, No. 3, p. 88, © American College of Medical Quality, 1991.

the importance of delivering this data to the end user (physicians and others) in a constructive manner, and providing effective alternatives for change. These alternatives might include the development of suggested clinical pathways for selected diagnoses; the implementation of specific policies or guidelines that monitor selected diagnostics, treatments, or procedures; or an intensified concurrent utilization review process that focuses on the appropriateness and effectiveness of the treatment plan. Positive change can be facilitated through computer-generated order entry systems. Such systems include "real time" feedback education screens that provide friendly reminders of the costs and indications for certain tests, or information regarding the appropriate utilization of antibiotics.

In step five of this process, medical staff input is continually elicited and conclusions are reinforced through ongoing physician education and monitoring.

CASE STUDY I: ORTHOPEDICS

When we first began our pilot studies, we elected to perform an in-depth study on one surgical diagnosis and one medical diagnosis. Because a preliminary study had already been conducted in the orthopedics department, and because of the high interest and enthusiasm of this particular group, we conducted our first comprehensive study on major joint procedures. Table 6–3 gives an example of our first data sort, examining DRGs 209–212 by number of cases, average length of stay, total gross revenues (charges), and charges as they accrue in the individual resource cost centers. Room charges represent charges for all board, care, and nursing; pharmacy charges represent all charges allocated to pharmacy, laboratory charges for lab services, and so on. The selection and categorization of each resource cost center is arbitrary, depending on the diagnosis selected and the areas earmarked for study. Table 6–4 examines the same group of diagnoses and resource utilization by individual physician.

The next level of analysis focuses on the individual resource cost centers to explore potential areas for improvement. Room

Table 6–3 DRGs 209–212 Major Joint Procedures

Diagnosis-Related Group (DRG) Summary Averages, 1987 (Before Study)

Charge/Patient, $

DRG No.*	Patients, no.	Average Length of Stay, days	Average Age, years	Gross Revenue	Room	Pharmacy	Laboratory	Surgery	Physical Therapy	Central Services	X-ray	Other Ancillary Charges
209	129	10.56	66	17,756	5,878	1,036	733	7,381	633	1,158	267	670
210	48	11.71	71	16,302	6,762	1,340	1,492	3,186	586	1,085	798	1,053
211	15	8.93	35	11,022	4,906	973	397	2,953	379	795	372	247
212	19	4.68	9	7,421	2,693	539	263	2,985	89	319	279	254
Total/Average	211	10.18	60	16,016	5,723	1,056	839	5,716	556	1,040	396	690

*DRGs 209–212 refer to Major Joint Procedures.

Source: Reprinted from The Western Journal of Medicine, Vol. 154, No. 2, p. 177, with permission of the California Medical Association, © 1991.

Table 6–4 DRGs 209–212 Physician Summary

Physician Summary Averages, 1987

Charge/Patient, $

Attending Physician	Patients, no.	Average Length of Stay, days	Average Age, years	Gross Revenue	Room	Pharmacy	Laboratory	Surgery	Physical Therapy	Central Services	X-ray	Other Ancillary Charges
1	2	9.00	70	17,444	4,924	807	950	7,337	618	1,076	218	1,514
2	15	8.87	59	15,881	5,042	1,157	896	6,170	545	1,000	487	584
3	2	6.00	31	6,256	3,299	395	84	2,187	0	245	0	46
4	10	10.80	69	17,416	6,153	1,397	886	6,342	599	1,176	255	608
5	6	10.00	77	15,451	5,909	991	1,337	4,168	574	842	774	856
6	51	10.27	64	17,310	5,652	990	771	7,151	610	1,196	288	652
7	14	9.21	59	12,964	5,155	846	615	4,085	497	819	436	511
8	9	16.44	66	22,693	9,251	1,635	1,224	5,924	1,109	1,506	789	1,255
9	15	10.73	62	19,050	6,261	1,357	1,072	7,106	519	1,739	299	697
10	1	6.00	78	9,135	3,300	161	414	3,091	336	552	810	471
11	28	9.29	57	14,297	5,111	860	587	5,456	516	937	287	543
12	14	6.86	15	11,292	4,039	750	388	4,908	210	498	305	194
13	12	9.50	62	14,312	5,284	972	802	4,754	480	836	522	662
14	3	14.33	68	20,267	7,937	1,063	1,785	6,223	637	1,152	593	877
15	11	11.18	62	16,227	6,150	1,148	719	5,186	505	894	474	1,151
16	7	13.57	83	19,779	8,316	1,628	1,959	3,167	775	1,231	906	1,797
17	8	11.13	62	13,903	6,075	1,277	1,007	3,483	607	514	382	558
18	1	12.00	74	19,411	7,425	916	1,629	5,479	588	1,933	367	1,074
19	1	11.00	80	15,728	5,775	481	590	7,199	511	832	0	340
20	1	5.00	42	9,184	3,015	505	486	4,294	231	301	173	179
Total/Average	211	10.18	60	16,016	5,723	1,056	839	5,716	556	1,040	396	690

Source: Reprinted from *The Western Journal of Medicine*, Vol. 154, No. 2, p. 178, with permission of the California Medical Association, © 1991.

charges would be affected by length of stay. In the laboratory, efficiencies could be gained by using a hemogram rather than a CBC, and a Type & Screen rather than a Type & Cross. In the pharmacy, judicious use of antibiotics and analgesics could improve efficiency. More judicious use of physical therapy services could improve efficiency in this category.

Table 6–5 gives a breakdown of the surgical cost center, including charges for time in surgery, anesthesia, recovery room, prostheses, and surgical supplies. When we looked at opportunities for improvement in this cost center, we noticed a striking degree of variation in the use of orthopedic prostheses. We were prompted to ask questions such as whether there was a need to use a $6,000 custom prosthesis if the standard $3,000 prosthesis would provide the same clinical result. This information was discussed with the chairpersons, selected individuals, and nurses of the orthopedics

Table 6–5 Surgical Cost Center

Surgery Summary of Diagnosis-Related Group 209, Hip and Knee Procedures, by Attending Physician
Surgery Charges Breakdown, Charge/Patient, $

Physician	Patients, No.	Total Surgery Charge/Patient, $	Surgery	Anesthesia	Recovery Room	Prosthesis	Tray/Pack/ Supply
1	2	7,337	2,229	423	575	3,278	831
2	10	7,285	3,044	438	399	2,694	711
3	0	0	0	0	0	0	0
4	9	6,581	2,421	398	328	2,612	821
5	1	6,382	1,720	351	361	3,132	818
6	42	7,949	3,039	448	436	3,109	918
7	6	5,882	1,838	360	255	2,573	856
8	5	7,441	2,657	407	403	3,103	871
9	12	7,912	2,301	458	287	3,501	1,366
10	0	0	0	0	0	0	0
11	18	6,999	2,619	379	374	2,782	845
12	4	9,392	4,464	464	346	3,565	553
13	6	6,759	2,468	353	223	2,902	813
14	2	8,034	4,588	433	336	3,810	772
15	7	6,375	1,830	340	424	2,946	834
16	1	6,418	2,055	445	305	2,950	663
17	2	6,933	2,542	320	347	2,935	789
18	1	5,479	1,540	220	401	2,675	643
19	1	7,199	2,263	370	442	3,770	354
20	0	0	0	0	0	0	0
Total/Average	129	7,381	2,719	414	378	2,985	886

Source: Reprinted from *The Western Journal of Medicine*, Vol. 154, No. 2, p. 178, with permission of the California Medical Association, © 1991.

department, and presented at the departmental meeting. Prior to the meeting, each physician in the department received a cover letter explaining the upcoming agenda. Included in this letter was a statement of purpose, a list of basic economic terms, and a confidential, nonidentified listing of each physician's profile as compared to his or her peers (Table 6–6).

The presentation began with an explanation of basic hospital economics and performance, and was followed by a discussion of the aggregate departmental profile data (see Table 6–7). It was stressed that the intention of our project was to exchange information in a constructive way, with the purpose of improving the overall process of care, and that this was not an accusation directed at any individual physician. In an effort to generate more group discussion, a break-even analysis graph was presented to illustrate the financial impact of services provided (see Figure 6–2). The top line indicates the total charges as accrued on a daily basis. Since surgery was performed on day one, the charges on the first day start with a high dollar value. The horizontal line represents the average net reimbursement received from all payers. The dotted line gives costs based on ratio of cost to charges.

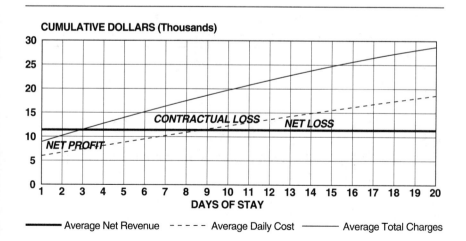

Figure 6–2 Total Hips: Break-Even Analysis.

Table 6-6 DRG 209 Physician Summary

INPATIENT

Attending Physician	Cases	Avg Age, years	Avg LOS, days	Gross Revenue Per Case	Room Revenue Average	Pharmacy Revenue Average	Surgery Revenue Average	Lab Revenue Average	Phys Thpy Revenue Average	Central Service Revenue Average	X-ray Revenue Average	Remaining Ancillary Revenue Average
A	10	68	11.0	20,268	5,643	1,056	10,024	910	477	946	318	894
B	24	76	10.5	23,037	5,931	1,475	9,642	1,440	620	1,848	370	1,711
C	21	65	9.8	21,014	5,457	1,367	9,964	983	578	1,762	303	600
D	9	72	11.4	21,510	6,000	1,725	8,331	1,478	764	1,967	265	980
E	6	77	8.5	17,519	4,383	709	9,705	743	511	824	215	429
F	61	60	9.3	21,038	4,736	1,464	10,464	805	581	1,691	229	1,068
G	8	74	7.8	17,129	3,699	1,482	8,398	955	487	1,149	290	669
H	11	76	11.9	28,443	8,485	2,284	8,490	2,465	725	2,193	994	2,807
I	21	67	10.2	22,184	5,361	1,222	11,625	879	658	1,238	136	1,065
J	5	73	16.0	24,441	9,025	1,655	4,364	3,349	892	2,473	740	1,943
K	18	69	10.0	20,642	6,021	1,429	8,450	1,229	552	1,880	390	691
L	5	80	8.0	20,600	3,665	4,419	10,032	609	399	1,233	184	59
McNamara	15	73	7.9	18,694	3,814	994	10,234	633	498	1,496	197	828
N	18	71	8.4	16,990	4,170	649	9,453	528	479	1,038	193	480
O	12	72	8.9	19,933	4,584	1,327	9,295	856	591	1,515	268	1,497
P	5	71	7.0	18,160	3,970	932	9,986	1,296	187	1,237	85	467
Q	17	78	8.9	16,597	4,632	919	7,845	836	496	825	271	773
R	10	76	9.8	20,335	5,891	1,001	9,375	890	464	1,698	283	733
S	6	69	10.0	18,936	5,350	737	9,947	919	640	748	312	283
T	8	72	9.8	20,501	5,319	1,747	9,758	1,323	526	856	150	822
U	5	59	5.0	15,126	1,880	620	9,987	674	154	1,382	303	126
DRG 209 Average	295	68	9.6	20,635	5,150	1,327	9,761	993	569	1,531	284	1,020

Contractual loss indicates the difference between costs and charges, though it represents a "paper loss." Net profit and net loss, however, represent the real difference between revenues received and costs incurred. In order to maximize the net profit section of the graph, the cost line can be moved to the left by reducing length of stay. In our meeting, one of the orthopedic surgeons suggested that we prepare the patient for earlier transfer to the Skilled Nursing Facility (SNF). He suggested that this could be facilitated by explaining to the family during the preoperative interview that the patient would be referred to the SNF earlier in the course of his or her rehabilitative therapy. Earlier mobilization to a lower level of care would be of primary economic benefit for patients covered by Medicare or other per-case reimbursement schedules, as well as patients covered under capitation.

The second way of maximizing net profit is to reduce unnecessary testing and procedures. Does every patient with a fractured hip need a computed tomographic (CT) scan or magnetic resonance imaging (MRI)?[63] This has particular implications for patients covered by Medicare and other per-case reimbursement schedules, and for patients covered by capitation and per diem payment schedules, which provide no additional reimbursement for services rendered. For our hospital, the latter three payer categories account for almost 75 percent of inpatient admissions.

Since our initial orthopedic presentation, we have been engaged in continuous monitoring of utilization patterns and are following up with physician education programs. Our published studies showed, after one year, an average 15 percent improvement in reduction of charges when comparing one-year results of the pre- and postintervention group, and reports show that efficiencies gained in these areas have been maintained.[64-66] The results are presented in Table 6–7.

CASE STUDY II: CONGESTIVE HEART FAILURE

Congestive heart failure represents the number one medical diagnosis among Medicare patients. Most hospitals are struggling

Table 6-7 Orthopedic Study Results

Orthopedic Diagnosis–Related Group (DRG)
Financial Trend Analysis of an Inlier Population, 1987 and 1988

Population and Services	Hospital Charge 1987	1988†	% Change From 1987	Population and Services	Hospital Charge 1987	1988†	% Change From 1987
Total population				DRG 211 Hip/Femur§			
Patients, no	164	187	14.0	Patients, no	13	29	123.1
Average length of stay, d	10.1	8.7	-13.9	Average length of stay, d	10.6	8.7	-17.9
Average age, yr	64	70		Average age, yr	54	78	
Average charge per patient, $				Average charge per patient, $			
Total gross revenue	16,107	15,145	- 6.0	Total gross revenue	12,254	12,275	0.2
Pharmacy	1,051	937	-10.8	Pharmacy	873	857	- 1.8
Surgery	5,771	5,926	2.7	Surgery	3,001	3,069	2.3
Laboratory	985	858	-12.9	Laboratory	520	924	77.7
Physical therapy	564	521	- 7.6	Physical therapy	596	462	-22.5
Central service	1,027	856	-16.7	Central service	560	755	34.8
X-ray	398	408	2.5	X-ray	535	668	24.9
DRG 209 Major Joint Procedure				DRG 212 Hip/Femur‖			
Patients, no	117	116	- 0.9	Patients, no	4	5	25.0
Average length of stay, d	10	8.5	-15.0	Average length of stay, d	8.5	8	- 5.9
Average age, yr	66	67		Average age, yr	11	8	
Average charge per patient, $				Average charge per patient, $			
Total gross revenue	17,188	16,513	- 3.9	Total gross revenue	9,600	10,066	4.9
Pharmacy	958	956	- 0.2	Pharmacy	597	501	-16.1
Surgery	7,377	7,725	4.7	Surgery	2,655	3,258	22.7
Laboratory	835	711	-14.9	Laboratory	427	446	4.4
Physical therapy	602	559	- 7.1	Physical therapy	189	168	-11.1
Central service	1,140	896	-21.4	Central service	360	511	41.9
X-ray	247	242	- 2.0	X-ray	356	567	59.3
DRG 210 Hip/Femur‡							
Patients, no	30	37	23.3				
Average length of stay, d	10.5	9.4	-10.5				
Average age, yr	72	82					
Average charge per patient, $							
Total gross revenue	13,721	13,972	1.8				
Pharmacy	963	1,012	5.1				
Surgery	2,775	2,929	5.5				
Laboratory	1,283	1,339	4.4				
Physical therapy	507	506	- 0.2				
Central service	756	869	14.9				
X-ray	744	712	- 4.3				

*Inlier population is defined as those patients with a length of stay ± 1 standard deviation from the average.

†Charges are adjusted for price increases between 1987 and 1988.

‡Hip and femur procedures except major joint procedures, in patients 18 years and older, with complications or comorbidity.

§Hip and femur procedures except major joint procedures, in patients 18 years and older, with complications or comorbidity.

‖Hip and femur procedures except major joint procedures, in patients aged 0 to 17 years.

Source: Reprinted from *The Western Journal of Medicine,* Vol. 154, No. 2, p. 180, with permission of The California Medical Association, © 1991.

due to revenues averaging less than 50 percent of charges for this particular diagnosis.

As with our orthopedics case study, we presented diagnosis and physician-specific data on congestive heart failure to members of the department of medicine of our hospital. See Tables 6–8 and 6–9 for examples of data aggregates in these areas. Again, we looked for opportunities for efficiency improvement by analyzing each individual resource cost center. Unlike a surgical diagnosis, in which most of the costs are related to the surgical cost center, the majority of costs in a medical diagnosis are evenly distributed among the ancillary cost centers. In fact, our estimates show that 50 percent of patient charges are a direct result of physician-ordered diagnostic and therapeutic services.[67] Costs related to room services are not only a reflection of length of stay, but also actual level of care. How quickly is the patient transferred from coronary care (if admitted to the coronary care unit [CCU]) to a transitional unit or the floor? We felt that there was an overutilization in the laboratory center of LDH isoenzymes that have essentially been superseded by CPK isoenzymes. Could oximetry effectively replace frequent blood gas determinations?

Therapeutically, we found that more aggressive diuretic therapy and use of other cardiac agents had a significant effect on total length of stay. Diagnostically, we had to consider if every patient needed a repeat echocardiogram, treadmill, or thallium scan, particularly if they just received one as an outpatient or for admission. The potential cost savings from bypassing tests that do not contribute to improved patient outcome are palpable.

The physicians in our hospital's department of medicine were also presented with a break-even analysis graph (Figure 6-3). At first glance, it appears to be similar to the graph on total hips, except for two major differences. First, there is a difference in break-even points—five days, compared to nine. It may be easy to reduce a length of stay of nine days to seven or eight, but reducing it from five days to three or four poses a greater challenge. There is also a difference in patterns of resource consumption. In the orthopedic example the costs are highest the first day because surgery was performed. In a medical diagnosis, the costs accrue gradually and are more evenly distributed among all the ancillary resource cost centers.

Table 6–8 DRG 127 Congestive Heart Failure

Individual Case Summary

Individual Cases*	LOS Days	Age, yr	Gross Revenue	Net Revenue	Operating Costs	Profit/ Loss	Variable Costs	Contribution Margin	Pharmacy Charges	RT/PF Charges	X-ray Charges	Lab Charges	EKG Charges	Room Charges	Other Charges
1	3	56	6,671	2,460	4,436	(1,976)	1,932	528	506	95	269	1,325	410	3,850	216
2	7	54	12,370	4,270	8,531	(4,261)	3,776	494	530	493	373	2,579	733	7,400	262
3	24	89	23,510	19,600	15,522	4,158	6,562	12,118	1,881	3,144	688	3,300	174	12,220	2,103
4	40	71	81,904	32,880	56,506	(23,706)	25,635	7,166	7,434	1,742	713	6,353	133	52,740	12,789
5	9	67	16,354	7,435	11,493	(4,058)	5,065	2,369	1,287	394	460	1,471	485	11,025	1,232
6	10	68	12,153	5,971	6,737	(776)	1,682	4,288	1,174	1,612	73	2,456	485	5,750	603
7	11	57	13,580	9,020	7,276	1,744	1,883	7,137	1,426	1,581	217	3,578	64	6,050	664
8	5	85	13,150	4,100	7,898	(3,798)	3,441	659	803	1,959	401	2,291	625	6,125	946
Total cases (171)	7.03 (avg)	73 (avg)	11,810 (avg)	6,575 (avg)	7,835 (avg)	(1,260) (avg)	3,393 (avg)	3,182 (avg)	830 (avg)	994 (avg)	294 (avg)	1,974 (avg)	317 (avg)	6,598 (avg)	803 (avg)

*Individual cases: representative case examples DRG 127; LOS: length of stay; gross revenue: based on hospital charges; net revenue: based on anticipated payments (adjusted for payer mix); operating costs: based on total (allocated) costs; profit/loss: derived from net revenue–operating costs; variable costs: indicate the additional cost of performing; contribution margin: derived from net revenue–variable cost; resource centers: pharmacy, respiratory therapy/pulmonary function, X-ray, laboratory, EKG (noninvasive lab), room, and remaining ancillary services.

Source: Reprinted from Rosenstein, A., "Utilization review: Health economics and cost-effective management," in *Quality Assurance and Utilization Review,* Vol. 16, No. 3, p. 89, © the American College of Medical Quality, 1991.

Table 6–9 DRG 127 Congestive Heart Failure: Physician Summary

Physician Case Summary

Physician ID#	Total Cases	Average LOS, days	Pharmacy Average Charge	RT/PF Average Charge	X-ray Average Charge	Laboratory Average Charge	EKG Average Charge	Average Gross Revenue	Average Net Revenue	Average Operating Costs	Profit/ Loss	Average Variable Costs	Average Contribution Margin
A	4	8.8	1,711	1,233	415	2,539	423	18,024	10,274	14,767	(4,493)	6,247	4,027
B	2	7.0	1,126	480	344	1,969	109	14,484	9,503	11,706	(2,203)	5,192	4,311
C	1	11.0	2,440	3,107	352	5,812	599	28,852	9,229	26,323	(17,094)	12,001	(2,772)
D	3	7.0	552	693	288	1,818	717	9,953	7,509	7,975	(465)	2,878	4,631
E	6	6.2	645	472	292	2,264	367	11,717	5,906	10,100	(4,194)	4,447	1,459
F	4	6.5	758	1,031	297	2,360	464	11,888	7,059	9,617	(2,588)	4,072	2,987
G	5	4.6	524	739	278	1,409	250	7,683	3,910	6,771	(2,861)	2,825	1,085
H	1	5.0	370	25	112	1,685	144	6,752	6,267	5,194	1,074	1,728	4,540

Source: Reprinted from Rosenstein, A., "Utilization review: Health economics and cost-effective management," in *Quality Assurance and Utilization Review*, Vol. 16, No. 3, p. 89, © the American College of Medical Quality, 1991

In attempting to maximize the net profit portion of the graph, one possibility is to reduce costs by shortening length of stay, thus moving the costs line to the left. However, we believe it is possible to have greater success at costs reduction by improving efficiency of care and reducing unnecessary testing and procedures—thus moving the cost line down. By following such guidelines, the process of care is improved not only for this one diagnosis, but there is also a positive, "trickle-over" effect on all diagnoses within the department.[68,69]

OUTCOME MANAGEMENT: THE FUTURE

Our present plan is to present department-specific information to all 23 clinical department chairpersons following the format presented in the preceding section.[70] We have organized a resource management team that includes members from administration; nursing; finance; contracting; information systems; ancillary department managers; utilization management; quality assurance; infection control; discharge planning; risk management; and other key departments in an effort to provide a collabo-

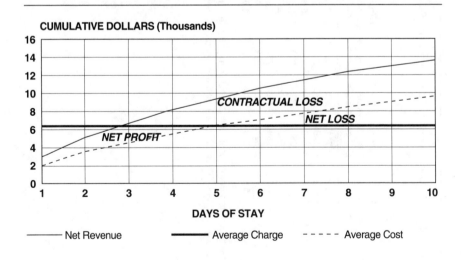

Figure 6–3 Heart Failure: Break-Even Analysis

rative framework for improving the process of care. Data from all departments will be collected and the resource management paradigm applied. Collectively, we refer to the implementation of these tools as Outcomes Measurement.[71]

We also plan to evaluate patients' functional and psychological perception of the health care intervention through use of patient surveys and questionnaires. This data will then be organized and integrated into a format to be delivered to both the medical staff and hospital departments in an effort to improve the process, quality, and cost-efficiency of care.

CONCLUSION

Today, there is an unprecedented pressure on the physician and health care organizations to provide quantifiable evidence of health care quality and cost-efficiency. Government agencies and business coalitions are actively collecting information on the cost and outcomes of medical care. Some reports provide hospital-to-hospital comparisons, while others, such as those recently produced in New York and Pennsylvania, provide physician-to-physician comparisons on the cost and outcome of procedures such as coronary artery bypass graft surgery. With public disclosure of outcomes data in combination with traditional marketplace forces, only the most efficient providers will prosper. Managed care organizations will likely try to enhance their competitiveness by reducing expenses through limiting overhead and streamlining operations.

The growing influence of managed care in the medical marketplace is placing new demands on physicians to maximize resource utilization. The managed care industry will employ several strategies to gain physician cooperation, including—but not limited to—financial incentives for high quality cost-effective practices. Physicians can also expect to see the increased use of practice guidelines, critical pathways, and clinical protocols. Managed care organizations are also rapidly enhancing their ability to gather data on the cost and quality of the care delivered. These data will provide feedback on practice patterns for both group practices and individual physicians. Physicians must be comfortable with the techniques and methods of quality assessment and cost-effective analysis in order to assist these organizations with meaningful interpretation of these data.

We have found from our experience in the hospital setting that medical resource management works. The tools employed are well within the range of most hospitals and managed care organizations. As more organizations gain large database capabilities, we project that medical resource management, with an eye toward outcome measurement, will be increasingly relied upon. A working knowledge of the principles of cost-effective analysis can go far in taking the mystery out of seemingly daunting cost containment strategies such as medical resource management. On a smaller but no less significant scale, it can also help us interpret studies cited in the literature, and perhaps inspire the application of some of these principles to our daily practices.

Physicians cannot be expected to adapt overnight to the plethora of reforms being imposed, nor obtain all the knowledge needed to effectively negotiate in this new environment. Only with time, and education by and for the profession can the ideal of cost-effective and quality health care be realized.

REFERENCES

1. Hornrook MC, Berki SE. Practice mode and payment method: effects on use, costs, quality, and access. *Med Care.* 1985; 23:484–511.

2. Yelin EH, Shearn MA, Epstein WV. Health outcomes for a chronic disease in prepaid group practic and fee for service settings: the case of rheumatoid arthritis. *Med Care.* 1986; 24:236–247.

3. Brook RH, Kamberg CJ, Lohr KN, Goldberg GA, Keeler EB, Newhouse JP. Quality of ambulatory care: epidemiology and comparison by insurance status and income. *Med Care.* 1990;28:392–433.

4. Udvarhelyi IS, Jennison K, Phillips RS, Epstein AM. Comparison of the quality of ambulatory care for fee-for-service and prepaid patients. *Ann Intern Med.* 1991;115: 394–400.

5. Murray JP, Greenfield S, Kaplan SH, Yano EM. Ambulatory testing for capitation and fee-for-service patients in the same practice setting: relationship to outcome. *Med Care.* 1992; 30: 252–261.

6. Epstein AM, Begg CB, McNeil BJ. The use of ambulatory testing in prepaid and fee-for-service group practices: relation to perceived profitability. *N Engl J Med.* 1986;314: 1089–1094.

7. Leape LL, Brennan TA, Laird N, et al. The nature of adverse events in hospitalized patients—results of the Harvard medical practice study II. *N Engl J Med.* 1991;324:377–384.

8. Clancy CM, Hillner BE. Physicians as gatekeepers: the impact of financial incentives. *Arch Intern Med.* 1989;149:917–920.

9. Johnson AN, Dowd B, Morris NE, Lurie N. Differences in inpatient resource use by type of health plan. *Inquiry.* 1989;26:388–398.

10. Manning WG, Leibowitz A, Goldberg GA, Rogers WH, Newhouse JP. A controlled trial of the effect of a prepaid group practice on use of services. *N Engl J Med.* 1984; 310:1505–1510.

11. Siu AL, Leibowitz A, Brook RH, Goldman NS, Lurie N, Newhouse JP. Use of the hospital in a randomized trial of prepaid care. *JAMA.* 1988;259:1343–1346.

12. Franks P, Clancy CM, Nutting PA. Sounding board: gatekeeper revisited—protecting patients from overtreatment. *N Engl J Med.* 1992;327:424–429.

13. Office of National Cost Estimates, Health Care Financing Administration. *1991–1992 Hospital Fact Book.* Sacramento, Calif: California Association of Hospitals and Health Systems;1992.

14. Faltermayer E. Let's really cure the health care system. *Fortune.* 1992;125:46–58.

15. Clark N. The high costs of dying. *The Wall Street Journal.* February 26, 1992.

16. Wasted health care dollars. *Consumer Reports.* 1992;57:435–448.

17. Woolhandler S, Himmelstein D. The deteriorating administrative efficiency of the U.S. health care system. *N Engl J Med.* 1991;324:1253–1258.

18. Chassin M, Kosecoff J, Park R, et al. Does inappropriate use explain geographic variations in the use of health care services? *JAMA.* 1987;258:2533–2537.

19. Winslow C, Solomon D, Chassin M, et al. The appropriateness of carotid endarterectomy. *N Engl J Med.* 1988;318:721–727.

20. Leape L, Rolla E, Solomon D. Does inappropriate use explain small area-variations in the use of health care services? *JAMA.* 1990;263:669–672.

21. Graboys T, Biegelsen B, Lambert S, Blatt C, Lowa B. Results of a second-opinion trial among patients recommended for coronary angiography. *JAMA.* 1992;268:2537–2540.

22. Pugh J, Frazier L, DeLong E, et al. Effect of daily charge feedback on inpatient charges and physician knowledge and behavior. *Arch Int Med.* 1989;149:426–429.

23. Morreim E. Fiscal scarcity and the inevitability of bedside monitoring. *Arch Int Med.* 1989;149:1012–1015.

24. Tierney W, Miller M, McDonald C. The effect on test ordering of informing physicians of the charges for outpatient diagnostic tests. *N Engl J Med.* 1990;322:1499–1504.

25. Shulkin DJ. Cost estimates of diagnostic procedures. *N Engl J Med.* 1988;919:1291.

26. Kassirer J. Our stubborn quest for diagnostic certainty—A cause of excessive testing? *N Engl J Med.* 1989;320:1489–1491.

27. Johnson H. Diminishing returns on the road to diagnostic certainty. *JAMA.* 1991; 265:2229–2231.

28. Kahn K, Rubinstein V, Draper D, Kosecoff J, et al. The effects of the DRG-based prospective payment system on quality of care for hospitalized medicare patients. *JAMA.* 1990;264:1953–1956.

29. Cooper H. Health care networks' attempts to cut costs are trimming patients' options. *The Wall Street Journal.* July 29, 1992;B1, B4.

30. Somers AR, Somers HM. A proposed framework for health and health care policies. *Inquiry.* 1977;14:115–170.

31. Shulkin DJ. Our army of doctors is waging war on health care costs. *Medical Economics.* June 1991:125–133.

32. Eisenberg JM, Nicklin D. Use of diagnostic services by physicians in community practice. *Med Care.* 1981;19:297–309.

33. Eisenberg JM, Williams SV. Cost containment and changing physicians' practice behavior: can the fox learn to guard the chicken coop? *JAMA.* 1981;246:2195–2201.

34. Cummings KM, Frisof KB, Long MJ, Hrynkiewich G. The effect of price information on physicians' test ordering behavior: ordering of diagnostic tests. *Med Care.* 1982; 20:293–301.

35. Loomas J, Anderson GM, Domnick-Pierre K, et al. Do practice guidelines guide practice? *N Engl J Med.* 1989;321:1306–1311.

36. Wathcel TJ, O'Sullivan P. Practice guidelines to reduce testing in the hospital. *J Gen Int Med.* 1990;5:335–341.

37. Rosenstein A. Do the right thing. *Federation of American Health System Review.* 1990;23:19–21.

38. Rosenstein A. Physician surplus—hospital vacancy strategic planning through mutual cooperation. *Health Care Strategic Management.* 1986;4:4–8.

39. Kendel P. Employers making use of price, quality data. *Modern Healthcare.* November 1991:42.

40. Meyer H. Some employers to select providers by outcomes. *AMA NEWS.* February 1990:48, 50.

41. Eisenberg J, Schwartz J, McCaslin F, et al. Substituting diagnostic services: new tests only partially replace older ones. *JAMA.* 1989;262:1196–1200.

42. Eisenberg JM. Clinical economics: economic analysis in medical care. Course Handout. American College of Physicians Annual Meeting, San Francisco, Calif: 1988.

43. Erban SB, Kinman JL, Schwartz JS. Routine use of prothrombin and partial thromboplastin times. *JAMA.* 1989;262:2428–2432.

44. Wennberg JE. Factors governing utilization of hospital services. *Hospital Practice.* September 1979:115–127.

45. Winslow CM, Solomon DH, Chassin MR, Kosecoff J, Merrick NJ, Brook RH. The appropriateness of carotid endartectomy. *N Engl J Med.* 1988;318:721–727.

46. Siegel DL, Edelstein PH, Nachamkin I. Inappropriate testing for diarrheal diseases in the hospital. *JAMA.* 1990;263:979–982.

47. Brown RT, Lossick JB, Mosure DJ, et al. Pharyngeal gonorrhea screening in adolescents. *Pediatrics.* 1989;84:623.

48. Deyo RA, Diehl AK, Rosenthal M. Reducing roentgenography use: can patient expectations be altered? *Arch Intern Med.* 1987;147:141–145.

49. Shulkin DJ, Detore AW. When laboratory tests are abnormal and the patient feels fine. *Hospital Practice.* July 1990:85–92.

50. Ravel R. *Clinical Laboratory Medicine: Clinical Applications of Laboratory Data.* 5th ed. Chicago, Ill: Year Book Medical;1989.

51. Feinstein AR. *Clinical Judgement.* Baltimore, MD: Williams & Wilkins Co.;1967.

52. Eddy DM. Clinical decision making: from theory to practice: the challenge. *JAMA.* 1990:263;287–290.

53. Hall WD. Urine sediment. In: Walker HK, Hall WD, Hurst JW, eds. *Clinical Methods: The History Physical and Laboratory Examinations.* Boston, MA: Butterworths;1976.

54. Somerville T, Murray W. Information yield from routine preoperative chest radiography and electrocardiography. *South Africa Medical Journal.* 1992;81:190–196.

55. Gagner M, Chiasson S. Preoperative chest x-ray films in elective surgery: a valid screening tool. *Canadian Journal of Surgery.* 1990;33:271–274.

56. Narr BJ, Hansen TR, Warner MA. Preoperative laboratory screening in healthy Mayo patients: cost-effective elimination of tests and unchanged outcomes. *Mayo Clin Proc.* 1991;66:155–159.

57. Sox H, ed. *Common Diagnostic Tests: Use and Interpretation.* Philadelphia, Pa: American College of Physicians;1990.

58. Rucker L, et al. Usefulness of screening chest roentgenograms in preoperative patients. *JAMA.* 1983;250:3209–3211.

59. Blery C, et al. Evaluation of a protocol for selective ordering of preoperative tests. *Lancet.* 1968;1:139–141.

60. Robins JA, Mushlin AI. Preoperative evaluation of the healthy patient. *Med Clin North Am.* 1979;63:1145–1156.

61. MacPherson DS, Snow R, Lofgren RP. Preoperative screening: value of previous tests. *Ann Inter Med.* 1990;113:969–973.

62. Rabkin SW, Horne JM. Preoperative electrocardiography: its cost-effectiveness in detecting abnormalities when a previous tracing exists. *Can Med Assoc J.* 1979;121:301–306.

63. Shulkin D, Rosenstein A, Mohlenbrock W. Quality care in a cost-conscious environment: treatment of a patient with a hip fracture. *Resident & Staff Physician.* 1992;38:33–39.

64. Stier M, Rosenstein A. Scrutiny of resource use can increase efficiency. *Health Care Financial Management.* November 1990:26–34.

65. Rosenstein A. Health resources management and physician control in a San Francisco, California hospital. *Western J Med.* 1991;154:175–181.

66. Rosenstein A. Attending physician and improvements in efficiency of medical operations. *Physician Executive Journal of Management.* 1991;17:33–37.

67. Rosenstein A. Cost saving due to lower utilization? *N Engl J Med.* 1991;325:739.

68. Rosenstein A. Health economics and resource management: a model for hospital efficiency. *Hospital Health Services Administration.* 1991;36:313–330.

69. Rosenstein A. Utilization review, health economics and cost-effective resource management. *Quality Assurance And Utilization Review.* 1991;6:1–2.

70. Rosenstein A. Overseeing cost-effectiveness in the provision of medical care. In: *Medical Management for Department Chiefs.* Tampa, Fla: The American College of Physician Executives;1992.

71. Rosenstein A, Miller L. Outcomes measurement: formula for success. *Clinical Outcomes.* 1992;3:2–3.

Editorial Commentary

David B. Nash

As the medical profession strives to maintain its balance in turbulent times, it is charged with spanning a chasm between what used to be, and what—virtually overnight—has become a new practice playing field. Not only must physicians learn to play by new rules; often, they must invent them. For example, physicians are expected to practice in a cost-effective manner, yet have few places to turn for learning how to do so.

Within the last two decades, the managed care laboratory has yielded numerous cost-containment and quality-assessment tools that have become de rigueur for the managed care physician, and the body of research continues to grow. One trend in this search for ever-improved ways of measuring cost and quality is the use of decision analysis techniques in planning and implementing medical interventions. Serving as a framework for decision analysis is the evaluation of economic implications on intervention strategies.[1] One need not be engaged in such state-of-the-art (and resource-intensive) efforts as decision analysis, however, to recognize the value of basic economic concepts in daily clinical practice.

David J. Shulkin and Alan H. Rosenstein are among the new generation of physicians dedicated to improving the cost-effectiveness of medical care. Drs. Shulkin and Rosenstein discuss how physicians, through the use of proven, practical strategies, can be catalysts for more cost-effective, quality care. Dr. Shulkin is a physician and the director of clinical outcomes assessment and quality management at the Hospital of the University of Pennsylvania in Philadelphia and a former Robert Wood Johnson Clinical Scholar. Dr. Rosenstein holds a comparable position at HBOC and Company, based in Atlanta and is responsible for providing feedback to physicians about their performance. Though hospital-based, the authors' strategies are targeted to the managed care setting.

First, the authors provide an overview of the forces contributing to the conundrum that is our current health care crisis. They emphasize the fact that economics alone do not drive health care costs. Often overlooked or underestimated in our search for a new, improved system are pervading social, legal, and educational norms that impact supply and demand. The authors' evaluation of the interrelationship between each set of factors gives us a clearer understanding of their role in fueling the vicious cycle of ever-spiraling costs, and stresses the necessity of addressing not only symptoms, but root causes, when formulating policy. The authors then discuss why these forces continue to act as barriers to implementing cost-effective care and, more importantly, how we can turn these barriers into bridges.

The authors then describe long-range cost-containment methods and strategies that go beyond current HMO tools such as utilization review and financial incentives. For example, they discuss how HMOs can instill in their physicians the ethos of cost-effective test ordering. They also present specific areas for cost-effective interventions, detailing a step-by-step, how-to process; and discuss the concept of outcome management, using case studies. For the "closet" economist, Drs. Shulkin and Rosenstein introduce the concept of cost-benefit analysis and its applications for the lay physician practice. We urge the uninitiated and skeptics alike to read on. To paraphrase Donald M. Berwick, MD, a leader in the field of Total Quality Management, acquiring these skills forms the essence of an organization's evolution toward continuous improvement.[2]

REFERENCES

1. Safran C, Phillips RS. Interventions to prevent readmission: the constraints of cost and efficacy. *Medical Care*. 1989;27(2):204–211.

2. Berwick DM. The double edge of knowledge. (Editorial.) *JAMA*. 1991;6:841–842.

Chapter 7

The Centers of Excellence Phenomena

Daniel Dragalin
Philip D. Goldstein

BACKGROUND

A *Center of Excellence* is commercially understood to be a pre-ferred institution whose staff has particular expertise in one or more specific procedures or therapies; that specific expertise is mar-keted by the institution in a focused fashion. In general, outcomes for the procedure or therapy are advertised as being state-of-the-art (with or without objective documentation). Various institutions have selected several areas for this kind of focused marketing, but targets are generally confined to relatively low-volume, but highly complex and costly procedures such as solid organ and bone mar-row transplantation and various cardiovascular surgeries.

The Centers of Excellence or specialized care center concept is a natural, targeted extension of the managed care concept. From a financial perspective, many institutions "bundle" professional and institutional fees for such procedures and therapies, offering a prospectively fixed price, generally with a significant discount over the individual retail components. From a clinical standpoint, the procedure or therapy is performed with above-average fre-quency by providers having above-average training and experi-ence in that focused area. The end result, theoretically, is the com-mercial offering of a service having a statistically above-average clinical outcome at a below-average package price. The goal of the supplying institution is to increase demand for these services from high-volume purchasers (insurance companies, managed care organizations, etc.) through preferred contracting. The goal of the purchaser is to obtain high quality services at discounted prices.

Whether the marketed services actually result in an optimal (state-of-the-art) outcome at a below-retail cost is institution specific. Both the clinical and the financial success of such programs are highly dependent on the diligence of the purchaser regarding institutional selection and the contracting process.

The Centers of Excellence concept has enjoyed relatively explosive growth over the past few years, reflecting increased concerns with medical costs, increased focus on managed care delivery systems, and increased purchaser scrutiny of quality of care. The major commercial insurance companies, the National Blue Cross and Blue Shield Association, many independent managed care organizations, and even a number of large employers have, over the past few years, signed preferred contracts with selected institutions to provide such services.

The Prudential Insurance Company of America calls these preferred institutions *Institutes of Quality* and The Metropolitan Insurance Company calls them *Centers of Quality*. The term used by Aetna is *Institutes of Excellence*, while The Travelers calls them *Specialty Care Institutes*. The Blues term them *National Transplant Networks* and CIGNA calls the product *LIFE SOURCE*. U.S. Healthcare calls them *The National Medical Transplantation Unit*.

The term *Centers of Excellence* was first copyrighted by Humana Health Plan to apply to individual hospitals in its network that specialize in selected procedures. The Honeywell Corporation then used the phrase to apply to a small network of preferred hospitals providing solid organ transplantation services to its employees. In the mid 1980s, Prudential expanded the concept into a large national procedure-specific preferred provider network offering bone marrow transplantation (allogenic and autologous) and solid organ transplantation services (heart, liver, lung, kidney, and eventually, kidney/pancreas). The concept was quickly adopted and expanded by other major payers, including the federal government. For a number of insurance carriers and provider organizations, the Centers of Excellence concept is now gradually being transformed. It is becoming a procedure-specific credentialing process that includes networks of institutions offering much more frequently performed procedures such as coronary artery bypass, coronary angioplasty, heart valve replacement, selected types of neurosurgery, and brain and spinal cord rehabilitation, to mention a few. Some managed care organizations are even applying this focused privileging process to diagnostic activities such as endoscopy and gastroscopy. Thus, procedure-specific credentialing, long used by hospitals in the staff privileging process, is rapidly becoming commercialized and integrated into managed care offerings as evidence of quality of care monitoring.

THE BIRTH OF A CONCEPT: HISTORY OF CENTERS OF EXCELLENCE

By 1987 and 1988, health care costs for most major employers had entered a seemingly endless spiral, increasing in the range of 15 percent to 25 percent annually. (See Figure 7–1.) Costs not only continued to climb but had become so unpredictable that it was extremely difficult for insurance companies to price offerings correctly. The year 1986 marked a return to underwriting losses last seen in 1983. The $1.5 billion total health insurance underwriting loss for 1986, however, paled in comparison to the $3.4 billion loss recorded in 1987. Nineteen eighty-eight produced record-breaking health care insurance losses in the area of $4.5 billion.

The Volume-Outcome Relationhip

By the latter half of the 1980s, increasing numbers of articles appeared, testifying to the waste, inefficiencies, and lack of

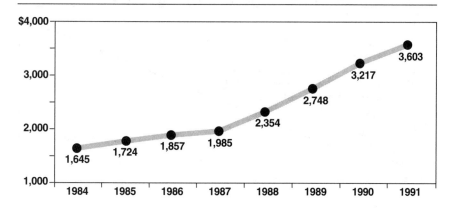

Figure 7–1 Average per Employee Health Cost 1984–1991. *Source:* A. Foster Higgins and Company Inc., Princeton, NJ, 1991.

documented quality of health care in the United States. Concomitantly, both the scientific and lay presses proposed various managed care delivery methodologies as the solution (at least partially) to the cost and quality issues in American medicine. In the search for documentable connections between enhanced quality of care and decreased costs, researchers began to examine more closely the relationship between clinical outcomes and procedural volume. In a report of the volume-outcome relationship written for the Office of Technology Assessment, Luft et al.[1] reviewed the abstracts of approximately 100 papers, eventually focusing on 13 surgical procedures and two medical diagnoses. The procedures ranged in complexity from appendectomies to abdominal aortic aneurysm repairs, and in expense from cardiac catheterization to total hip replacements. Solid organ transplantations were not included in the study.

The analysis was difficult due to varying methodologies within the individual studies, but the findings were generally consistent with the hypothesis that worse outcomes occur at lower volumes for selected procedures. Specifically, in studies of certain procedures and medical diagnoses (see Figure 7–2) a positive relationship was found between volume and outcome.

Luft et al. reasoned the "practice makes perfect" explanation of the volume-outcome relationship rests on the general notion that

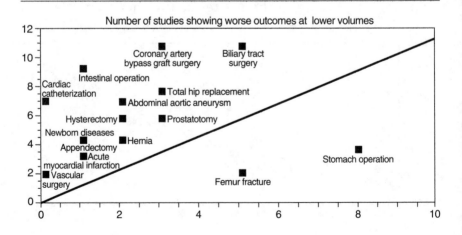

Figure 7–2 Volume Studies Reviewed by OTA. *Source:* Office of Technology Assessment, Washington, DC, 1988.

increased experience results in more finely developed skills and, therefore, in better outcomes. The surgeon who consistently performs many units of a specified procedure will maintain, or continue to improve, his or her skills, while the surgeon who performs few procedures will become progressively less proficient. Similarly, nursing and other staff who are more familiar with certain types of patients may become or remain more proficient in working with them. Higher volumes may also make it possible for hospitals to purchase specialized equipment for such patients.

The authors went on to postulate,

> Even if physician volume is most important, hospital volume is likely to play a role. For example, a hospital with several high-volume and several low-volume surgeons may develop monitoring methods and standard procedures for the staff that catch errors and institute corrective actions. Thus, a low-volume surgeon may be "protected" in a high-volume hospital. Likewise, a surgeon with a high volume across several institutions but low volumes in each may achieve good results.

Finally, in a sort of "academic disclaimer," the authors noted,

> Volume may not matter at all, but instead may serve as a marker for hospitals or physicians with special skills whose better-than-average performance attracts a disproportionate share of the referrals. This "selective-referral" hypothesis holds that any inverse relationship between volume and outcome arises from the attraction of more patients to physicians and hospitals with better outcomes.[1]

Figure 7–3, the hypothesized relationship between volume and outcome—first published in the Luft et al. analysis—became the subject of significant discussion in the growing search for clinical quality markers.

An additional, highly publicized study[2] evaluated the correlation between volume and mortality on five procedures performed in New York State hospitals in 1986. The procedures were cholecystectomy, coronary artery bypass, resection of abdominal aortic aneurysm, partial gastrectomy, and colectomy. The study confirmed that a statistically significant correlation existed between hospital and physician volume and outcome of the procedure.

A study by Laffel et al. also supported the hypothetical relationship between volume and outcome, at least for cardiac transplantation.[3] In a slight modification to the general belief, the authors put forth the compelling argument establishing a "threshold" number of procedures (at least for cardiac transplantation) necessary to reach optimal outcomes. Their findings suggest a relatively diminishing rate of outcome enhancement for institutions and surgeons performing beyond the required threshold number of procedures.

In summary, while far from definitive, these analyses provided substantial evidence that worse outcomes occur at lower volumes for the procedures and diagnoses studied.

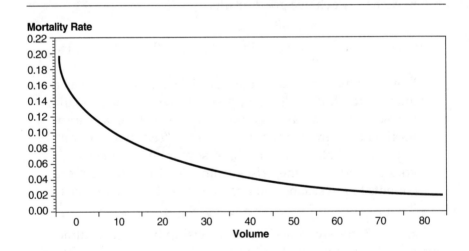

Figure 7–3 Relationship between Volume and Outcome. *Source:* Office of Technology Assessment, Washington, DC, 1988.

THE INITIAL TARGET—ORGAN TRANSPLANTATION

Organ transplantation, while costly, does not contribute significantly to overall private sector health insurance costs. (See Figure 7–4; Table 7–1.) The Hewitt consulting firm published an often-quoted analysis focusing on the factors responsible for continuing health care claims costs (see Figure 7–5). Most of the blame for cost increases is centered on cost-shifting from federal programs (33 percent), medical inflation (30 percent), utilization increases (20 percent), and technologic advances (8 percent). Catastrophic care is only assigned 10 percent of the blame; solid organ transplantation, AIDS, burns, and neonatal cases all occupy the catastrophic slice. Indeed, in the experience of most large commercial carriers, annual charges for solid organ transplantation account for less than 1 percent of total annual claims dollars.

Despite the relatively low aggregate expense for solid organ transplantation, the proliferation of transplantation centers, the limited donor organ supply, the literature on the volume-outcome hypothesis, the federal government focus on transplantation, and the "life-or-death" emotion surrounding organ transplantation, reimbursement decisions made transplantation a likely candidate for scrutiny.

During the latter half of the 1980s, there was heightened public awareness regarding the substantial increases in both the number

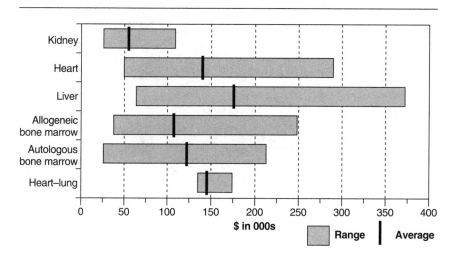

Figure 7–4 First–Year Expenses of Organ Transplants. *Source:* Health Insurance Association of America, Washington, DC.

Table 7-1 Average Cost Differentials

	Heart	Liver	Kidney
Retail	$127,000	$200,000	$70,000
Contract	$95,000	$145,750	$47,290

Source: The Prudential, Roseland, NJ, 1991.

of organ transplantation procedures performed (see Figure 7–6) and the number of centers offering transplantation programs (Figure 7–7). While the increase in the number of transplant procedures appeared to mirror the growth in programs, actual experience was dramatically different. In 1988, less than one-half of the heart transplant centers performed 12 or more heart transplant procedures. Seventeen performed no transplants and of the 113 that did perform transplants, 66 performed 10 or fewer procedures. There were also lung transplantation centers that did not perform any transplants in 1988 and, of the 208 kidney transplantation centers, 105 performed 25 or fewer procedures in 1988.

Organ Donor Availability

Organ donor availability in the late 1980s was not keeping pace with the improved surgery techniques and improved immuno-

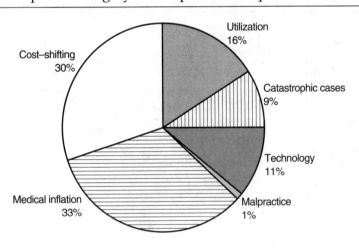

Figure 7–5 Factors Contributing to Increases in Annual Medical Benefit Costs. *Source:* Hewitt, New York. NY. 1993.

Number of procedures

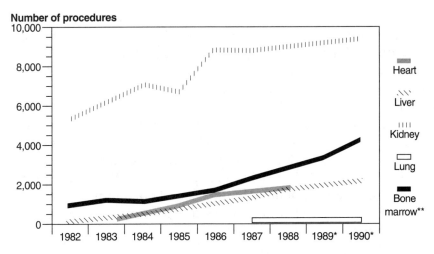

*Data for 1982–1988 are from the American Council on Transplantation, with the exception of 1988 bone marrow transplants, which are an M&R estimate. 1990 estimates are based on previous trends. M&R 1989 estimates are based on 1988 and 1990.

**1982–1986 bone marrow transplants reflect nonautologous transplants only, whereas 1987–1990 include autogolous transplants.

Figure 7–6 Annual Number of Selected Organ Transplants in the United States. *Source:* Milliman and Robertson, Los Angeles, CA, 1990.

November 1988 – October 1990

Number of procedures

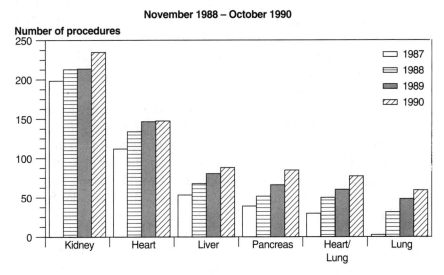

Figure 7–7 Number of Solid Organ Transplant Programs Registered with UNOS. *Source:* United Network for Organ Sharing, Chicago, IL, October 1990.

suppressive drug regimens that made organ transplantation a viable option for more patients. There had been only a modest growth in donor organ supply in the preceding years. On the premise that experience directly relates to outcomes for selective procedures, and that experience is enhanced by the volume of similar procedures performed, health care analysts concluded that continued proliferation of organ transplant programs in the face of marginal or no increases in available donor organs was not in the best interests of high quality medical care. Yet many institutions—because of decreasing occupancy (and therefore, falling profit margins) secondary to intense cost-containment pressures—were diversifying into services not previously offered; solid organ transplantation, cardiac surgery, mental health, and rehabilitation were prime targets.

Task Force on Organ Transplantation

Concurrent with (or as the result of) increasing public scrutiny of organ transplantation, and as a result of the enactment of the National Organ Transplantation Act of 1984, the federal government eventually commissioned the formation of the Task Force on Organ Transplantation to study organ transplants in the United States. Two major results were the formation of the United Network for Organ Sharing (UNOS) and the creation of regional organ procurement organizations with established quality guidelines for donor organ acquisition and sharing protocols.

Among the recommendations of the Task Force was the requirement that hospitals belong to UNOS. In order to belong to UNOS, hospitals were obliged to meet certain criteria relating to annual procedure volumes and outcomes for each organ transplant type. In 1988, UNOS published guidelines for transplant surgeon training, surgeon and hospital annual volumes, and revised survival thresholds for heart, liver, kidney, and pancreas transplants. The original UNOS membership criteria for heart transplantation rates were fairly aggressive for the time; a minimum of 12 transplants were required annually with a one-year graft survival rate of 73 percent and a 2-year graft survival rate of 65 percent. In addition,

UNOS established guidelines for donor selection and organ distribution. Any new program had two years to comply with UNOS membership criteria.

Two years earlier, in 1986, the Health Care Financing Administration (HCFA) had already determined that heart transplants should be eligible for Medicare reimbursement but reimbursement was limited to only those institutions with documented experience in successful procedure performance. In order to qualify as a Medicare heart transplant center, the hospital was required to have an established program that performed at least 12 transplants annually for the two years prior to application and achieved a one-year patient survival rate of at least 70 percent.

THE FIRST LARGE COMMERCIAL NETWORK

In 1987—one year before the publication of the Office of Technology Assessment analysis on procedural volumes and outcomes—the Prudential Insurance Company, the largest commercial carrier at that time, decided to establish a nationwide network of preferred institutions for heart, liver, and kidney transplantations. An earlier attempt to organize a national network of kidney stone lithotripsy centers had failed because of the unanticipated explosion in the number of lithotripters in the United States. Prudential believed that a successful preferred network focus on an individual procedure depended on the procedure or therapy having several characteristics:

- The procedure or therapy should be costly enough to justify the expense of both the selection and negotiation process, and the additional costs associated with transportation.
- There should be well-defined indicators of quality for the procedure or therapy that should be published in the scientific press; those indicators should reflect benchmarks for optimal (state-of-the-art) clinical results.
- All of the published quality indicators should be measurable.
- Published literature should reveal significant variations between institutions in the quality of clinical results for the procedure or therapy.

- There should be documented evidence that the clinical end-result was improvable with additional experience (institutional and/or provider).
- Institutions considered for admission to the network should be able to accept a significant volume of additional patients without compromising the quality of care.
- A significant net gain should be realized by the purchaser for diverting these selected patients to the preferred institutions.

Solid organ transplantation fit the bill. The medical literature was researched and studies were collected that demonstrated a relationship between specific experience (or medical practices) and optimal outcomes for the various types of organ transplantations. These experiences or practices were then codified (see Exhibit 7–1) into standards to be used as normative quality base-

Exhibit 7–1 Sample Quality Standards

Heart	Liver	Renal
■ The program must be at least 2 years old.	■ The program must be at least 2 years old.	■ The program must be at least 2 years old.
■ Each physician on the transplant team must have at least 1 year of training and 2 years of experience with transplants.	■ Each physician on the transplant team must have at least 1 year of training and 2 years of experience with transplants.	■ Each physician on the transplant team must have at least 1 year of training and 2 years of experience with transplants.
■ A minimum of 15 transplants must be performed annually.	■ A minimum of 12 transplants must be performed annually.	■ A minimum of 25 transplants must be performed annually.
■ The 1-year patient survival rate must be greater than 80–82%.	■ The 1-year patient survival rate must be greater than 77%.	■ The 1-year patient survival rate must be greater than 95–98%.
■ In conjunction with the heart transplant program, the institution must have an established cardiovascular surgical program and must perform: — A minimum of 250 open heart procedures annually. — A minimum of 500 cardiac catheterizations annually.		■ The 1-year graft survival rate must be greater than: — 70% for a living, related donor organs. — 65% for a cadeveric donor organ.

lines to "qualify" institutions or practitioners for network inclusion. A Request for Proposal (RFP) was drawn up and issued nationwide to over 300 institutions offering organ transplantation services. Approximately 50 percent of the institutions responded and approximately one-half of them met the standard quality criteria published in the medical literature. A number of the institutions meeting the quality criteria were then reapproached for financial bidding sessions. The Prudential objective was to negotiate a fixed-price, per-procedure contract with institutions having optimal clinical outcomes. All professional and institutional fees, preprocedure workups, laboratory testing and imaging, postprocedure monitoring, and possibly even the cost of complications were to be included in the package price.

At that time, most hospitals had not negotiated package prices with their staffs; accordingly, many were unable to quote a comprehensive fixed price combining both institutional and professional costs. In fact, almost one year elapsed prior to the completion of the national network because of pricing difficulties. The first national commercial solid organ transplantation network was completed in July 1988 and was quickly followed by the completion of an allogeneic bone marrow transplantation network in 1989.

At the time, the "retail" value of a heart transplantation (institutional, professional, and ancillary fees) was approximately $127,000; contracts were negotiated averaging prospective fixed-rate prices of $95,000, a 25 percent discount. Liver transplantations were "selling" for approximately $200,000; contracts were negotiated that averaged around $146,000—again—a substantial discount. Kidney transplantations "retailing" at $70,000 were negotiated, on the average, down to $47,000.

From a pricing perspective, negotiations were favorable for Prudential. For the first year of the network, 77 referrals were made to preferred institutions.

BENEFIT DESIGN

In general, most insurance carriers using the Centers of Excellence concept offer benefit enhancements as additional incentive to use preferred institutions. The trend for health care plans today is not to pay first-dollar coverage and to increase both the deductible and out-of-pocket responsibilities of the patient. In general, Centers of Excellence benefits cover 100 percent of eligible charges and waive the deductible. When the patient must travel to be seen by a preferred provider, travel expenses are fully reimbursed for both the patient and a companion (usually a family member). Reimbursement for hotel expenses and a daily living allowance are also provided for a selected companion as well as the patient, to ensure the patient has the necessary emotional support. The companion can also provide competent decision making and important information should the patient become incapacitated. Additionally, an insurance nurse case manager is generally assigned to monitor the patient (by phone) from the presurgical workup through the rehabilitation period to ensure that the administrative process flows smoothly.

Some of the benefits associated with Centers of Excellence packages, such as the transportation and lodging reimbursement for the patient and a companion, are not ordinarily associated with insurance coverage. The benefits, however, are similar to "extra-contractual benefits" often found in managed care systems and used in the case management of selected patients. One of the unique insurance coverage differences between indemnity insurance and managed care insurance (especially regarding self-funded plans of large employers) is the ability of the employer (or plan manager) to reimburse, at their discretion, for certain "convenience" expenses such as transportation, lodging, temporary custodial care, normally noncovered medical equipment, and so forth. This coverage often enables patients to take advantage of alternative settings and therapies that ultimately benefit both the patient (through enhanced care) and the employer (through cost savings generated from the avoidance of less effective traditionally covered care). This coverage flexibility, although it must be used judiciously to avoid violation of insurance regulation, is increasingly seen as a major enhancement of managed care systems in general, and Centers of Excellence programs in particular.

The *Institute of Quality* package was marketed within Prudential managed care organizations (health maintenance organizations

[HMOs] and preferred provider organizations [PPOs]) and within the traditional major medical insurance lines. Most employer clients with indemnity (nonmanaged) insurance who elected the package chose to enhance benefits for preferred institutions rather than reduce benefits for nonpreferred institutions. Accordingly, a number of benefit packages were created that increased hospital and surgical coverage and decreased deductibles for using the preferred institutions.

On the managed care side, it was difficult to legally mandate the use of preferred institutions. Federally qualified HMOs are obliged to provide "basic services," if they are available, in their own geographic service area. The Health Care Financing Administration (HCFA) considers most organ transplantations to be "basic services." Therefore, if a nonpreferred institution offers transplant services within the defined geographic area, the patient has the choice of using, without penalty, either the nonpreferred institution or a more remote preferred institution. Even PPOs, filed under state insurance laws, generally do not mandate the use of out-of-state institutions if institutions inside the state offer transplantation services—regardless of quality. Some states, however, are beginning to allow HMOs to mandate the use of preferred institutions, if the institutions are located in the organization's primary service area. For example, the Pennsylvania Department of Health has allowed Prudential to mandate the use of Philadelphia-based specialized center facilities for its HMO members. If, however, a Philadelphia-based, contracted tertiary hospital which is not a Center of Excellence offers the same service as a non-Philadelphia-based specialized center facility, the HMO may not mandate the use of the out-of-area center.

An additional benefit complication is the fact that, for most patients needing organ transplantation, the benefit plan "stop-loss" (out-of-pocket maximum) has already been met prior to the surgery. Thus, even for nonpreferred, out-of-network institutions, maximum benefits are due. In summary, whether in the indemnity or the managed care setting, financial influences are generally not the patient's deciding factor in using a Center of Excellence. The perceived quality of the institution itself is the deciding factor in most cases.

CURRENT NETWORKS

Less than a dozen commercially available national organ transplantation networks exist today. All the major commercial insurance carriers maintain multistate networks, as does the Blue Cross and Blue Shield Association and the HCFA. The number of institutions in each network varies, as depicted in Table 7–2. While approximately 80 institutions are members of one or more networks, less than a dozen are generally members of all networks:

1. University of Minnesota (heart, lung, kidney, heart-lung, bone marrow)
2. Cleveland Clinic (heart, liver, bone marrow)
3. University of California at Los Angeles (heart, liver, bone marrow, kidney)
4. Emory University Hospital, Atlanta (heart, liver, bone marrow, kidney)
5. Barnes Hospital at Washington University, St. Louis (heart, liver, bone marrow, kidney)
6. Baylor University Medical Center, Dallas (heart, liver, bone marrow, kidney)
7. Brigham and Women's Hospital, Boston (heart, lung, bone marrow)

Credentialing standards are reasonably uniform between networks; several networks maintain numerous and highly detailed

Table 7–2 Network Size

	Aetna	BC/BS	CIGNA	MET	Travelers	Prudential
No. of Institutions						
Heart	3	37	7	4	8	12
Liver	4	19	4	2	8	7
Kidney			1	10	1	16
Lung	1		3		1	5
Heart-lung			2		1	2
Pancreas				1		
Kidney/pancreas			2		1	
Bone marrow	2	31	2	3	8	7
Unduplicated Total	4	64	13	15	12	23

credentialing criteria. Common major criteria are detailed in Exhibit 7–1.

FUTURE DILEMMAS

A number of issues related to reimbursement for solid organ transplantation are increasingly being discussed within the insurance community. These issues deal with basic reimbursement policy:

- Should organ transplantations not yet conclusively proven to be effective be covered? For example, substantial controversy exists regarding the effectiveness of pancreas-only as opposed to pancreas/kidney transplantation.
- Should insurance companies pay for human hearts used as "bridges" to keep patients alive while a better donor match or stronger heart is sought?
- During the past decade, surgeons have performed some 2,000 double or triple organ transplants, mostly for severe diabetes, and over the past two years, three patients have been given four or five organs simultaneously. What should the reimbursement policy be for multiple-organ transplants in a society with a limited organ donor pool?
- Recently, physicians in a number of countries, including the United States, have given a portion or lobe of a parent's liver to a child with fatal liver disease; are such living donor transplant patients eligible for reimbursement?
- Cluster operations, generally involving people under age 49 with terminal cancer of the liver and bile ducts, involve removal of virtually all the organs and tissues in the upper abdomen— the liver, spleen, stomach, and small intestine; should these operations be reimbursed?
- What effect will FK 506 and its successors have on rejection? This is an experimental immunosuppressant from Japan with much less toxicity than cyclosporine; Syntex in California is experimenting with a similar drug—RS 61443.

These and other questions will become topics of substantial debate throughout the 1990s.

LESSONS LEARNED

Some valuable lessons were learned during the first few years of experience with the network. Given the explosive growth and commercialization of the Centers of Excellence concept, a number of physicians (especially those practicing in nonpreferred institutions) have expressed doubts about the claims of better outcomes in some preferred institutions. Confirmation of institutional claims of "excellence" in a given area is, of course, the responsibility of the purchaser; the selection criteria imposed by large commercial carriers is fairly exacting and remarkably similar between carriers. Unfortunately, many carriers remain unable to objectively demonstrate the clinical results over time. Surprisingly, many commercial insurers continue to market only the criteria used for institution selection and are not capable of providing data supporting the original claims of superior outcomes. Given the reputations of many of the selected institutions, such data will no doubt be produced eventually. However, at present, it remains the responsibility of a new purchaser to repeat due diligence in each new selection effort. Practicing physicians encouraged to refer patients to such institutions should explore, through the managed care plan, current institutional outcomes. For many procedures, overall institutional outcomes may change suddenly and dramatically. Changes in surgical teams may occur. Other changes may involve support personnel, procedural approaches, or introductions of new equipment or adjunctive therapies. Within a given institution, an aggregate measurement of outcome may appear favorable; however, in institutions with large numbers of specialists or specialist teams performing a given procedure, the indication is that outcome may vary widely. The hospital and community-based physician mix may contribute to the observed outcome variability.

One of the major sources of "savings" for organ transplantation is the result of candidates being declared ineligible for the procedure. Each preferred institution retains its own patient selection criteria and performs its own final evaluation of the candidate prior to surgery. Because of the limited donor organ supply, the final decision to transplant rests with the institution. This rigorous "appropriateness screening" serves as a sophisticated second surgical opinion, screening out candidates without sufficient organ function impairment, and candidates whose disease is judged too advanced for a transplant to reverse. Any candidate denied access by a preferred institution is allowed to obtain a second, and possibly even a third opinion from other preferred institutions. These external opinions significantly enhance the objectivity and ethical implications of the ultimate reimbursement decision (as well as increasing its legal defensibility).

In the managed care setting, a member's attitudes about the preferred network varies depending on how referral to a tertiary care center is presented by the physician (especially when travel is involved). Prudential found that commitment to the program by the plan medical director is particularly crucial.

In terms of legal ramifications, the selection of tertiary care centers based on quality of care and the subsequent "advertisement" of that quality unquestionably increases carrier liability. This is because of the patient's enhanced expectations when using the preferred center. Networks cannot simply be formed and forgotten—they must be continuously monitored. Legal consultation in the initial phases of network formation is indispensable.

NETWORKS IN DEVELOPMENT

Because of the explosion in the use of high dose chemotherapy and subsequent autologous bone marrow rescue for various types of cancer, many allogeneic bone marrow transplantation networks are being converted to autologous networks, and additional institutions are being added. Experimentation with peripheral stem cell rescue and the use of colony stimulating factors may prevent autologous networks from realizing expected volumes in the future.

Another highly viable area of extension for these networks is the area of cardiac surgery, including coronary artery bypass grafting, angioplasty, cardiac valve replacement, and pediatric cardiac surgery. The addition of these procedures to the Centers of Excellence concept moves the concept into a new dimension—that of local procedure-specific credentialing.

Hospitals with open heart surgery units are much more numerous than institutions offering organ transplant services. In a given metropolitan area, a dozen institutional choices may exist. Again, as for solid organ transplantation, definitive optimal outcomes exist (Exhibits 7–2 and 7–3). Additionally, the opportunity to negotiate discounted package prices is also present; coronary artery bypass grafting has an average "retail" value (1992) of approximately $37,000 (professional and institutional charges). However, it is possible to negotiate package prices for as little as $15,000 in selected institutions.

FUTURE TRENDS

The dilemma facing network managers in a managed care environment is that hospitals already in the general medical/surgical network may not qualify to offer these more specialized procedures and may therefore risk losing considerable market share. The network manager using procedure-specific credentialing at the local level may also risk losing discounts on other bed types if he or she attempts to separate out specialty procedures. Fortunately, market demand from large employer clients for procedure-specific outcome information may, appropriately, drive the

Exhibit 7–2 Percutaneous Transluminal Angioplasty Sample Minimum Criteria

- Annual volume, institution: 200 procedures
- Average volume—operator: 75 procedures
- Procedural mortality: 0.5–1.0%
- Nonfatal myocardial infarction: 4–5%
- Emergency CABG: 3–6%
- Type A success: 85%
- Type B success: 80%

Exhibit 7–3 Coronary Artery Bypass Grafting Sample Minimum Criteria

■ Annual volume: 250 procedures
■ Average length of stay: 8 days
■ In-hospital mortality: 3–5%
■ 5-year survival: 90–95%
■ 10-year reoperation: 10–12%
■ Internal mammary artery use predominance

decision toward optimal clinical outcomes rather than short-term cost savings or marketing considerations.

A few variations on the developmental theme are now occurring. The John Hancock Insurance Company has joined with a single provider and a pharmaceutical firm to develop a program to improve outcomes for sufferers of severe asthma. The National Jewish Center for Immunology and Respiratory Medicine is the provider and Schering-Plough Corporation is the pharmaceutical firm. The program will identify patterns of severe asthma within the Hancock book of business. Beneficiaries who have had repeat emergency admissions, frequent physician visits, and high medical use may be flown to National Jewish for evaluation. Asthma affects 12 million Americans, costing the health care system roughly $6.2 billion per year. Thirty percent of costs are generated by 2 percent of the patients.

A slightly different approach is being used by U.S. Healthcare, which is focusing on a number of diseases, rather than confining efforts to procedures. This large provider has identified specialists throughout the United States who deal with relatively uncommon but expensive chronic illnesses, such as multiple myeloma.

Additional procedures and therapies currently under consideration by a number of carriers for the development of procedure-specific preferred networks include:

* corneal transplantation
* selected neurosurgical procedures
* cochlear treatments

- cranial/facial reconstructive surgery
- head and spinal cord injury rehabilitation
- treatment of multiple myeloma
- treatment of refractory asthmatic cases
- mitral valve replacement surgery
- adult arteriovenous (AV) malformations of the brain
- treatment of sarcoma
- total surgical replacement of the aorta

An additional twist on the theme is the emergence of "carve-out" products. A carve-out is a separately packaged and priced component of an otherwise integrated managed care delivery system. For example, mental health services (with or without substance abuse rehabilitation services), pharmacy services, or selected specialty services all have been packaged and sold by vendors as stand-alone services. Thus, an employer is able to purchase mental health services from one company, pharmacy services from another, and so forth.

The many carve-out mental health and substance abuse programs in the market today could also be considered another form of procedure-specific credentialing and a further step in increasing specialization of managed care credentialing processes. An approximate half-dozen managed care firms targeting the national market and many more firms targeting local and regional markets have emerged to provide carve-out mental health and substance abuse rehabilitation services to mostly large, self-funded employers. These focused managed programs can be used with an indemnity plan—thus making mental health the only "managed" component of the benefit design—or as a replacement for the mental health portion of a managed care plan. Many corporate benefit managers believe that the mental health portion of their managed care plan is less developed and less effective than the medical/surgical portion. Managed care administrators and medical directors often tend to focus on refinement and enhancement of the medical/surgical aspects of their system and are often less aggressive with the mental health and substance abuse aspects. Thus, it is often not difficult for firms specializing in mental health services to convince employers to replace those portions with specialized and focused plans.

While mental health carve-outs with focused monitoring have indeed enhanced managed care programs in the past, there now appears to be a move toward a reintegration of medical/surgical services with mental health and substance abuse services. As managed care plans have matured, administrators—under competitive pressures from mental health service firms—have concentrated on the set of services within their own plan, making them far more competitive. From a clinical standpoint, it is somewhat difficult to separate the two sets of services. Prescription profiling of primary care physicians in managed care plans with separate mental health and substance abuse carve-outs reflects a relatively high frequency prescription of psychotropic drugs. This fact is not lost on benefit managers and health care consultants who are beginning to argue for reintegrated systems.

Another form of carve-out tangentially related to the Centers of Excellence concept is in the pharmaceutical area. Differing from the mental health product in that it is primarily based on software and pharmacy discounts rather than enhanced service, pharmacy product growth has been especially fostered by point-of-service (POS) plans. POS plans are similar to conventional PPOs in that the beneficiary receives enhanced benefits for using preferred services and reduced benefits for using nonpreferred services. A major difference between a POS plan and a PPO is that the in-network portion is much more tightly medically managed (similar to an HMO). In pharmacy carve-outs, preferred pharmacies are equipped with software allowing the pharmacist to check beneficiary eligibility, pharmaceutical contractual stipulations, and the presence or absence of selective benefits such as generic incentive programs or formularies. As with mental health products, the growing sophistication of managed care programs in the pharmaceutical field may cause pharmacy carve-outs to be a short-lived phenomenon.

CONCLUSION: IMPACT ON THE PRACTICING PHYSICIAN

For many employers and insurers, the Centers of Excellence concept has proven to be one of the few hard pieces of evidence linking enhanced quality of care with diminished health care costs. For many providers participating in such networks, the Center of Excellence label has quite successfully been used as a marketing tool to draw even further volume.

Selective procedure-specific contracting is becoming increasingly commonplace. It remains to be seen whether managed care networks will refine general credentialing standards to the level of individual privileging for member physicians. Many health care experts view the specialized care center approach as the forerunner of procedure-specific credentialing for individual physicians in the managed care setting.

Another critical conclusion that can be drawn from the increasing focus on credentialing and outcomes inherent in the Centers of Excellence concept is that practicing physicians will increasingly be held accountable for results by managed care programs. Outcomes-oriented data currently required by specialized care programs are similar to the data being generated on practicing physicians in a number of managed care programs. While physician credentialing efforts in managed care programs have always been relatively extensive, the more aggressive systems are creating practice profiles of their physician members. These profiles include prescribing practice patterns, ancillary test ordering, hospitalization of chronic patients, hospital adverse occurrence monitoring, compliance with preventive care protocols, and overall patient satisfaction. All are currently being documented by some of the more advanced managed care systems. Individual physician financial incentives are being set by performance in the various areas of medical practice. In some managed care systems, these performance incentives can have a 30 to 40 percent impact on physician income.

With increasing endorsement and encouragement of managed care programs in both the public and private sectors, both primary care physicians and specialists can, in the near future, anticipate individual outcome-oriented monitoring similar to that of the specialized care programs. As with Center of Excellence credentialing and monitoring, it is not unreasonable to anticipate substantially increased scrutiny on procedure- and disease-specific physician experience against comparative norms. Also, it is not unreasonable to anticipate a change from the use of local norms to national norms. This codification of "best practices" based on outcome and the emerging linkage between optimal practices and outcomes, credentialing, and financial incentives will undoubtedly improve the overall practice of medicine.

REFERENCES

1. Luft HS, Gernick DW, Mark D, McPhee SJ, Tetreault J. *Volume of Services in Hospitals or Performed by Physicians.* Rockville, MD: Office of Technology Assessment; 1988.

2. Hannan EL, Kilburn H, Lukacik G, Shields EP. Adult open-heart surgery in New York State. an analysis of risk factors and hospital mortality rates. *JAMA.* 1990; 264:2768–2774.

3. Laffel GL, Barnett AI, Finkelstein S, Kaye MP. The relation between experience and outcome in heart transplantation. *N Engl J Med.* 1992;327:1220–1225.

Editorial Commentary

Susan L. Howell
David B. Nash

The concerted push toward managed care begun in the 1970s launched a multitude of HMO "hybrids," each of which has had varying success in surviving the storms of a capricious market and health care reform efforts. Among these managed care offspring, the Centers of Excellence phenomena are proving to be tenacious indeed.

A Center of Excellence, or specialized care center, is a generic term for an institution or group of providers who perform a specialized procedure at a discounted (prospectively fixed) price to payers, who in turn pass this low cost on to patients. The Centers concept was given a jumpstart in the 1980s with the publication of several major studies that found a positive relationship between volume and outcome. Thus, the current popularity of the Centers of Excellence model is due to its promise of enhanced quality of care as well as decreased costs.

The authors, Daniel Dragalin, MD, and Philip D. Goldstein, MD, have prepared a chapter describing the Centers of Excellence programs, which many managed care companies now sponsor. Dr. Dragalin is a principal with Towers-Perrin, a large health care consulting firm in New York, and Dr. Goldstein is an executive with a large, independent practice association in suburban Philadelphia, Pennsylvania. Drs. Dragalin and Goldstein began by giving us an overarching view of the ingredients comprising these "phenomena" and led us through the history of the Center of Excellence movement—beginning with the trend to integrate managed care with organ transplantation, spearheaded by Prudential—to the present day. The authors also gave us an enlighted look at the "lessons learned" by Prudential in their role of pioneer in this new field. We learn the types of procedures typically offered by specialized care centers and are introduced to other new procedures on the horizon. The authors address new developments in the managed care/specialized care center arena, including mental health and pharmaceutical "cut-outs."

As is emphasized throughout this book, the role of data collection and management information systems in the managed care setting is a paramount tool to help monitor and enhance quality; this is particularly true for specialized care centers, whose viability (i.e., marketability) depends so heavily on its ability to deliver a quality product at low cost. Increasingly, insurers demand routine, outcomes-oriented data from member providers. The authors discuss how managed care organizations use hospital-specific data in developing specialized care centers, the use of data in practice profiling and facilitating efficiency in hospital processes, and the impact on quality.

Lastly, the authors hypothesize on the future of the specialized care center setting and the implications for physicians. They suggest that we may soon see a more widespread utilization of tools such as procedure-specific credentialing and practice profiling—currently employed by Centers at the individual physician level. Given the success of the Centers, which is showing no signs of abating, it is not surprising they are being viewed by many as a bellwether within the managed health care arena.

Chapter 8

Understanding Your Managed Care Practice: The Critical Role of Case Mix Systems

Norbert Goldfield

With the new administration's emphasis on managed care, case mix systems will assume heightened importance as tools to help physicians understand resource consumption and aspects of quality. The case mix tools described in this chapter will significantly enhance the ability of physicians to provide value-enhanced services to their managed care organization (MCO). In particular, reliable and valid case mix systems will be needed to risk-adjust the capitation rate for the increasingly large numbers of patients enrolled in competing MCOs. While MCOs have focused their greatest cost control efforts on the outpatient sector, they spend more than half of the health premium dollar on inpatient services. Thus, it is critical that managed care physicians become aggressive in utilizing claims-based tools that shed light on both inpatient and outpatient services.

This chapter will

1. summarize the salient characteristics of the clinical case mix classification systems most frequently utilized in managed care systems
2. illustrate the use of these classification systems in MCOs
3. detail recent research trends in clinical case mix classification systems

After reading this chapter, managed care physicians will understand

1. the theoretical underpinnings of the most commonly used ambulatory and inpatient case mix systems

2. how different case mix systems can be used for either utilization management or quality improvement
3. the economic and quality-of-care incentives that can be engendered utilizing case mix systems

The specific systems discussed in this chapter are Diagnosis Related Groups (DRGs); various DRG systems adjusted for patient severity; and Ambulatory Patient Groups (APGs).

INTRODUCTION

Given the relative rapidity of their "institutionalization" into the health care system, it is hard to believe that DRGs have been used by Medicare for hospital reimbursement for less than ten years. Case mix systems have had a significant impact on physician practice patterns.[1] This impact has grown from the systems' original application as a hospital payment system for inpatient care to one used by MCOs for contracting, severity-adjusted physician profiling, and identification of areas of quality improvement for both hospitals and MCOs. Over the past decade, this increase in functionality has been facilitated by significant refinement in DRG case mix systems and the development of case mix systems relevant to the ambulatory sector.

The implementation of inpatient case mix systems for payment purposes has had a significant impact on other aspects of the health care system. Of great significance, DRG use by Medicare for payment has, among other factors, led to an explosion in outpatient services.[2] The rapid development of outpatient services has prompted a managerial and regulatory demand for the development of outpatient case mix systems such as APGs.[3] The dramatic rise in costs attributable to the outpatient sector has prompted Congress to mandate the Health Care Financing Administration (HCFA) to develop and propose for implementation the extension of prospective payment to the outpatient sector.[3]

Thus, in 1993, health professionals and institutions can derive significant benefits from ambulatory and inpatient case mix systems. These case mix systems are useful in the best sense of a much over-used term: *quality improvement*. That is, classification systems such as DRGs and APGs can be used to break down the very complex health care system into basic "building blocks." Each "block" is unique in that it contains diagnoses and/or procedures that are similar from both a clinical and resource consumption point of view. Assembled into a health care scheme for an individual or group of patients, these blocks can be used to better understand resource consumption and quality considerations of either the inpatient and/or outpatient aspects of an entire health system.

These building blocks can also be used to "incentivize" appropriate resource use. This is how the DRGs are currently used by Medicare. However, institutions are increasingly utilizing quality improvement techniques to understand how to better use existing resources, thus maximizing reimbursement per DRG. In both cases, institutions look to quality improvement in an effort to provide better health care and lower costs.

It should be emphasized that without significant medical leadership interest, capability, and support, case mix systems are valueless. DRGs and APGs are merely tools; they do not, in themselves, provide answers nor do they constitute action. Case mix tools are important but they are only part of the medical director's armory. They can be effectively utilized within a context of overall institutional commitment to true quality improvement. In fact, once that commitment exists, follow-through will be difficult without use of case mix tools.

HISTORY OF CASE MIX SYSTEMS

Our current commitment to quality improvement can be traced back to Eugene Codman, a surgeon at Massachusetts General Hospital in Boston, Massachusetts. While much of his work has been viewed as the precursor to our understanding quality of care outcomes, it can also be viewed as anticipatory of DRGs and APGs. In his path-breaking article appropriately entitled *The Product of a Hospital*, Codman says, "It would be supposed that in the annual reports of hospitals some account of their products would be found. To a certain extent this is true, but often much of the material in an annual report is but a mere account of money subscribed and the proportionate amounts which are spent on the different departments."[4] (p196)

When Dr. Codman presented his data on outcomes of care to his colleagues at the 1917 conference of the American College of Surgeons in New York City, they responded by burning his report in the fireplace of the meeting hall. Case mix research remained at this level until the late 1960s, when Fetter, Thompson, Averill, and other researchers at Yale University began to adopt a fresh look at this issue: "In 1967 a group of physicians at our local university hospital asked for help with a problem of utilization review. At the time, two years after the advent of the Medicare program, all hospitals were required to operate a program of utilization review and quality assurance as a condition for receiving Medicare funds. The physicians asked whether industrial methods of cost and quality control could be adapted and applied to the hospital industry."[5]

Sixteen years later DRGs were implemented by the HCFA as a payment tool for hospitalized Medicare patients. (The developers of the DRGs did not initially envision that they would be utilized for payment purposes.) In response to the request by the physicians at Yale-New Haven Hospital, Fetter and his colleagues tried to develop a system that would be useful for managerial purposes. In constructing this management tool, the developers were guided by several considerations:

1. Class definitions based on information routinely collected on hospital abstracts
2. Manageable number of classes
3. Similar patterns of resource intensity within a given class
4. Similar types of patients in a given class from a clinical perspective.[5]

This organizational approach resulted in the DRGs' implementation in early 1980s. The Medicare inpatient prospective payment system (PPS) has been successful in controlling the growth of Medicare inpatient care expenditures. In 1990, these expenditures were $18 billion less per year than estimated in the early 1980s.[6] Because of the success of the inpatient PPS, it was natural that the federal government would look to an outpatient equivalent to inpatient PPS when faced with the staggering rise in outpatient services.

AMBULATORY CASE MIX SYSTEMS

The cost and quantity of ambulatory care services has exploded over the past ten years. The reasons for this dramatic rise are manifold and include clinical, regulatory, and competitive factors. Analysts point to the implementation of Medicare DRGs in 1983 as a key change leading to the rise in demand for these services.[7] Other important factors include changing technology and the rise in managed care services. While regulators and corporations demanded a better handle on inpatient hospital costs in the 1980s, these same groups are now shifting their attention to ambulatory care. The rise in ambulatory services has prompted an effort on the part of payers, clinicians, and health services researchers to better understand the content of the ambulatory encounter.

It is particularly important that the conceptual issues pertaining to ambulatory case mix systems be fully understood in order to accurately measure resource consumption and quality of care for managed care services. Thus, for example, the most important hurdle managed care systems face in both pricing and quality of care decisions is the development of an effective case mix adjustment of the capitation rate for managed care enrollees. The inadequacy of the tools currently used to adjust these rates is a fundamental stumbling block to a complete commitment to managed care. When an effective system is developed, it will enable MCOs and physicians to confidently compare and contrast the quality of care and cost of service rendered.

There are two keys to developing a valid ambulatory classification for payment and quality improvement procedures such as physician profiling: accurate understanding of resource consumption and clinical coherence. Whether the ambulatory case mix system (ACMS) is used for visits or episodes, for quality management or payment, it is imperative that the different classes statistically reflect differences in resource consumption. Herein lies the fundamental challenge in developing a reliable and valid ACMS, as outpatient services are so variegated. The complexity of ambulatory services also increases the challenge of making an ACMS clinically cogent, a necessity if it is to be embraced by health professionals.

Components of an ACMS

There can be up to three parts to an ACMS: the classification system; the "bundling" algorithm of the classes (which describes the entire ambulatory encounter); and, if the ACMS is to be used for reimbursement, a payment computation. Some ACMs consist only of a classification system. In the classification system, each member of a class consumes similar resources. Each class purports to describe similar ambulatory encounters, from either a resource consumption or clinical cogency perspective. Ambulatory Visit Groups and Diagnosis Clusters are examples of this type of ACMS. Other ACMS combine or bundle different classes that together describe the ambulatory episode or visit. The bundling logic depends on clinical and nonclinical factors such as cost and frequency of test performances. Thus a plain film might represent a service that could be bundled into the primary services provided during the encounter. APGs are examples of this type of ACMS. If the system is to be utilized for payment, the third component of the ACMS—payment computation—needs to be developed. That is, the resources consumed in each class or combination of classes needs to be translated into a payment amount. APGs were specifically developed to be utilized as a payment system.

Challenges in Creating an ACMS

There are two main obstacles to creating an ACMS: the complexity of ambulatory encounters and problems inherent in current coding systems. Ambulatory encounters are complex for both clinical and organizational reasons. Ambulatory care constitutes a service that is frequently provided in the face of poorly understood clinical conditions.[8] A large percentage of ambulatory visits involve a sign, symptom, or finding for which, at the completion of the ambulatory visit, the clinician has not decided on a firm diagnosis.[9] The poorly understood nature of many conditions seen in ambulatory services is exacerbated by a poor understanding of patient motivations for seeking medical care.[10] As a consequence, ambulatory care patients often complain of symptoms (such as back pain) for which medical science has not developed effective treatment, and often there is a difference in opinion between the physician and the patient as to whether the condition was fully treated. Thus, the inadequate medical understanding of back pain results in significant difficulties in creating a clinically cogent class of uniform resource intensity for a symptom that is one of the most frequent reasons for ambulatory encounters.

There are two aspects to the administrative complexity of ambulatory care. From a sheer geographic perspective, both the patient and physician are typically confronted with a myriad of possible institutions from which to obtain needed services. Many of these institutions are located in widely disparate locations. Also, unlike the inpatient setting in which a physician and nurse typically coordinate all aspects of patient care within the hospital's four walls, there is usually no such coordination in the ambulatory care arena. Even if the patient is enrolled in an HMO that provides managed care, there typically is little true coordination of care between the physician's office, laboratory, and radiology facility—often located miles apart. The diffuse nature of ambulatory care adds significantly to the difficulty in packaging the content of ambulatory encounters into one category.

In contrast to ambulatory services, there is little difficulty in defining beginning and end points for inpatient care. When a patient remains overnight in the hospital, his or her entire existence occurs within those four walls. The content of inpatient care is thus more easily measured than that of ambulatory care, in which there is a constant interplay between the physician's office, home, and other loci.

Another challenge in developing an ACMS is pinpointing what defines a "new" ambulatory care patient. This critical issue is one that bridges clinical and organizational concerns. Several of the visit-based systems use "new" vs. "old" patient as a classifying variable. This variable is utilized because of the assumption that a "new" patient consumes a different quantity of resources than an "old" patient. However, the validity of this distinction becomes suspect when one attempts to define "new." A patient can be new to the primary provider, the provider seeing the patient on that occasion, or to the institution. "Newness" may represent a structural element of the doctor-patient encounter that superficially appears to be a reasonable predictor of resource consumption but that, on further examination, cannot be clearly nor reliably specified.

The inadequacy of current coding systems further complicates the already difficult task of developing an ACMS. Two coding systems are in common use in the United States today: International Classification of Disease, 9th Edition, United States version (ICD–9–CM) and Current Procedures and Terminology–4 (CPT–4). CPT–4 is mainly office-based and is procedures-oriented. ICD–9–CM is primarily oriented toward inpatient care.

In summary, ambulatory encounters are poorly understood and difficult to classify. As detailed in the preceding discussion, some of the primary reasons for this include:

- deficiencies in clinical knowledge
- varied patient responses to the same poorly understood clinical condition
- disparate settings from which the patient can choose to obtain ambulatory services
- minimal coordination, in this era of managed care, of the varied services that patients may obtain
- difficulty in defining a "new" ambulatory patient
- facility-specific variables such as queing (time in line for appointments)
- inadequacy of coding systems for describing ambulatory services

APGs

Under contract to the HCFA, APGs were developed as an ACMS that could be utilized for the prospective payment of ambulatory care.[3] The APGs are a patient classification scheme designed to explain the amount and type of resources used in an ambulatory visit. Patients in each APG have similar clinical characteristics, resource use, and costs. The process of formulating the APGs was highly iterative, involving statistical results from historical data combined with clinical judgment. The end result of this process is a clinically consistent group of patient classes that are homogenous in terms of resource use. There are 145 procedure APGs, 80 medical APGs, and 72 ancillary service APGs, totaling 297 APGs. The APGs as currently constructed describe the complete range of services provided in the outpatient setting. The APGs can form the basic building blocks for a visit-based outpatient PPS and provide a flexible structure enabling managed care organizations to use the APGs for contracting and physician profiling purposes.

APGs are a significant departure from DRGs in several ways:

1. The initial classification variable for APGs is whether or not a significant procedure was performed. Normally, a significant procedure is scheduled, constitutes the reason for the visit, and dominates the time and resources expended during the visit. Examples of significant procedure APGs include carpal tunnel repair and stress tests. A medical visit occurred if a provider was seen and a significant procedure was not performed. Examples of medical APGs include hypertension, headache, and hematological malignancy.
2. There can be only one DRG per hospital stay. There can be more than one APG per ambulatory encounter.
3. DRGs use ICD–9–CM for classification. APGs utilize both ICD–9–CM and CPT–4.

Payment for Ambulatory Services Using APGs

In constructing the APGs, the developers decided that a visit-based PPS for ambulatory care had three components: the patient classification scheme; a significant procedure consolidation and ancillary packaging process; and payment computation and discounting.

When a patient has multiple significant procedures, some of the procedures may require minimal additional time or resources. Significant procedure consolidation refers to the consolidation of multiple related significant procedure APGs into a single APG for the purpose of determining payment. For example, if both a simple repair and complex repair (two separate APGs) are coded on a patient bill, only the complex skin incision will be used in the APG payment computation.

A patient with a significant procedure or a medical visit may have ancillary services performed as part of the visit. Ancillary packaging refers to the inclusion into the APG payment rate of certain ancillary services for a significant procedure or medical visit. A uniform list was developed of ancillary APGs that are always packaged into a significant procedure or medical visit. Examples of packaged APGs include APGs for plain films and electrocardiograms. Packaging is a critical part of the APG system. Without it there would be no economic incentive to appropriately utilize services such as complete blood cell counts and plain films. These services may appear to be inconsequential. However, these small ticket items constitute almost 60 percent of all claims submitted to Medicare for outpatient services.

When multiple unrelated significant procedures are performed or when the same ancillary service is performed multiple times, a discounting of the APG payment is applied. Discounting refers to a reduction in the standard payment rate for an APG. Discounting recognizes that the marginal cost of providing a second procedure during a single visit is less than the cost of providing the procedure by itself.

Though APGs were initially developed for the payment purposes, they can be used in several aspects of the quality improvement process.

Monitoring Quality of Care Utilizing APGs

APGs can be further used to improve quality in three ways. First, APGs can assist Continuous Quality Improvement (CQI) efforts. For example, an institution attempting to document the results of a CQI intervention in the area of vaccination can effectively utilize APGs that combine a large number of vaccine-related CPT codes into one of three groups, based on resource cost of the three groups. Thus, it can profile vaccination rates more effectively using three groups in lieu of innumerable CPT codes.

APGs also can identify potential areas of inappropriate ambulatory care resources utilization. For example, one might track—utilizing control charts—the use of ancillaries such as electrocardiograms, plain films, and inexpensive laboratory tests (each of which constitutes an APG) for elective procedures such as upper gastrointestinal endoscopies, herniorrhaphies, and cataract removals. These results could be profiled by physician, ambulatory care setting, or other organizational variables. It should be emphasized that aberrant results provided by APGs should not be utilized as definitive measures of inappropriate utilization. Rather, if a large database is available, the results could be tracked over time using a control chart. If results become "out of control," a CQI team could determine the sources for the aberrant data.

Lastly, APGs provide decision makers—particularly those in managed care—with an accurate picture of the types of patients covered by their primary care physicians. Use of this information for the assignment of primary care physician panels of patients could, in turn, result in increased provider and patient satisfaction.

From the example below, medical directors of group practice plans and PPOs will learn that:

1. It is easier to contract for services utilizing a smaller number of APGs than utilizing the large number of codes in the CPT manual.
2. The APG groups are clinically cogent.
3. One can track the frequency with which procedures, for example, are performed with much greater ease utilizing APGs.

Case Study. Blue Cross and Blue Shield of Northern California is in its second year of utilizing significant procedure APGs for contracting purposes in its managed care organizations, particularly its preferred provider organizations (PPOs). Both Blue Cross/Blue Shield (BC/BS) and individual hospitals found it much easier to contract on the basis of a small number of clinically meaningful categories such as APGs, rather than deal with a large number of CPT codes. Payment for ancillary services is not included at the present time. Personnel in charge of contracting at BC/BS are presently working with the most common significant procedure APGs consisting of more than 80 percent of all procedures (surgery and otherwise) performed in an outpatient (hospital and ambulatory surgery center) setting. BC/BS personnel were able to much more efficiently contract for and price out services utilizing APGs in lieu of individual CPT codes.

Feedback from health care institutions has been positive from both administrators and clinicians, indicating that the APGs can be differentiated on both a clinical and resource consumption basis.* Ancillary services could have been included if there was an interest in encouraging appropriate use of frequently ordered inexpensive items.

DRGs AND THEIR APPLICATION TO MANAGED CARE

DRGs have become a universal language that hospitals, managed care organizations, and insurance companies utilize in discussing—to use Codman's term—the "product of a hospital."[4] DRGs can help managed care physicians to identify areas in need of quality improvement. Most managed care organizations contract with hospitals on the basis of either simplistic combinations of DRGs, per diems, or capitation. This approach assumes that the hospital and its full-time personnel are responsible for understanding the factors leading to increased resource consumption and poor quality. Managed care physicians will increasingly be asked to become involved in hospital operations in order to contribute to the quality improvement process for their patients.

Utilizing claims-based case mix systems, such as the DRG refinements described in this chapter, will enable managed care physicians to work with their administrative colleagues in explaining resource consumption variations and quality of care,

---

*Information provided by Robert Langley, Blue Cross/Blue Shield of Northern California.

and identification of the best contracting opportunities. Many hospitals and managed care companies currently utilize severity-adjusted DRGs. Interest in severity-adjusted tools has risen dramatically, particuarly with the arrival of such claims-based tools as All Patient Refined (APR)-DRGs, which are much less labor intensive than medical records-based tools, such as Medisgrps and Computerized Severity of Illness (CSI). Several states have mandated the use of APR-DRGs or Medisgrps for comparative purposes.

There are four critical parts to understanding the structure of DRGs:

1. organ system
2. distinction between surgical and medical procedure
3. categorization of procedures and a categorization of medical problems
4. other indicators that differentiate processes of care

When the DRG definitions were originally developed in the 1970s, the DRGs were intended to describe all types of patients seen in the acute care hospital. Unfortunately, conventional analyses by DRG can provide an insufficient and incomplete comparison of cost, length of stay (LOS), and mortality of data. When the efficiency of providers showing higher costs or lengths of stay is questioned, the likely response is "my patients are sicker." A more refined classification is needed to identify patients who have different resource needs and outcomes. In the mid-1980s, researchers began looking at ways to account for these differences based on DRG classification. Age, co-morbidities, and complications constitute a level 4 indicator that modifies DRG assignment. Physician panels examined each ICD–9–CM code to identify codes that constituted comorbidities and complications according to the following algorithm: a condition that in combination with a specific principal diagnosis would cause an increase in length of stay by at least one day in at least 75% of the patients.[5] This effort to identify complications and/or comorbidities resulted in a list of approximately 1,000 ICD–9–CM codes. Virtually this same list of codes is still used by HCFA.

Before dicussing DRG variants currently used throughout the world, it is important to specify a lexicon of the confusing terminology pertaining to DRGs:

HCFA DRGs. Implemented in 1983, these DRGs are used by the HCFA for hospital reimbursement on a prospective basis for Medicare patients. They are updated annually. A contract for their enhancement is provided to researchers at 3M/HIS with final decisions resting with researchers and policymakers within the HCFA. Considerable effort has been extended to refine the DRGs to account for complexity without having to examine the medical record. The following DRG refinements, all using claims-based information, have occurred since the initial implementation of the HCFA DRGs.

AP-DRGs. All Patient (AP)-DRGs have been used by New York State since 1987 for prospective payment for all non-Medicare inpatient services provided in the state. They have been specifically developed to account for cost variance for all ages and types of patients. Thus the National Association of Children's Hospitals and Related Institutions (NACHRI) provides input into the formation of these DRGs as they pertain to pediatric populations. They are updated annually with input provided by researchers at 3M/HIS and reseachers/policymakers at the New York State Department of Health (NYDH). Currently, the states of New York, Massachusetts, Maine, and Washington utilize some form of AP-DRGs for payment or budget reconciliation purposes. Numerous Medicaid programs and many foreign countries utilize the HCFA or AP-DRGs for internal budgeting purposes.

Yale-Refined DRGs. In the mid-1980s, researchers developing the original DRGs subdivided the HCFA DRGs into subclasses (3 for medical and 4 for surgical) based on differences in resource consumption resulting from the presence of specific comorbidities and complications. This research, funded by the HCFA, has formed the basis for many of the currently available severity systems that purport to adjust DRGs for severity.

APR-DRGs. APR-DRGs are used by hospitals and governmental organizations to examine issues of complexity or severity within a DRG. They are applicable to all ages and types of patients. They have not been used for payment or budgeting purposes, because many of the APR-DRG categories are too small to set a payment weight. Four classes are created for both medical and surgical DRGs. Classes represent distinct differences between patients in both resource consumption and severity of illness.* Voluntary Hospitals of America (VHA), the largest hospital chain in the United States, has recently made available APR-DRGs in a large number of its hospitals.

Management Objectives of Refining DRGs for Severity

The concept of severity is even more misunderstood than the term *quality improvement*. In discussing severity, several terms, often used interchangeably, should be defined. It is critical that the applied research community clearly distinguish among these terms.

Severity of illness refers to the relative levels of loss of function and mortality experienced by patients with a particular disease. *Treatment difficulty* refers to the patient management problems that an illness presents to the health care provider. Such management problems are associated with illnesses lacking a clear pattern of symptoms, illnesses requiring sophisticated and technically difficult procedures, and illnesses requiring close monitoring and supervision. *Need for intervention* relates to the severity of illness that lack of immediate or continuing care would produce. *Resource intensity* or *severity of service* refers to the relative volume and types of diagnostic, therapeutic, and bed services used in the management of a particular illness.

Inpatient Case Mix Systems

Researchers have refined DRG technologies in an effort to delineate and better understand the reasons for measuring case mix. Hospital administrators are most interested in a severity adjusted case mix system that provides improved statistical explanation of resource consumption variance within a DRG category. In contrast, managed care physicians are most likely concerned with the relationship between treatment pattern differences and severity of the patient's illness. In deciding whether to concentrate on intensity of resource consumption or severity of illness, it is important to question who will most likely benefit from an improved explanation of resource consumption variance—the medical staff,

---

*Material drawn from 3M/HIS.

administrative leadership, or other members of the health care team? Both the medical and administrative leadership need to decide which dependent variable (costs, length of stay, mortality, or complications) needs to be better explained.

The intended audience for DRG refinements such as APR-DRGs is both the administrative and medical leadership of the managed care setting. The APR-DRGs attempt to explain the variance in severity of illness and intensity of service for patients enrolled in a managed care plan, utilizing information derived from a claims form. By bridging these two diverse audiences, the APR-DRGs shed light on cost differences between categories that have been adjusted for severity. While variance in cost may represent a variance in severity of illness in 80 percent of the cases, there are notable exceptions. Acknowledgment of these exceptions will hopefully clarify the severity of illness debate, which unfortunately has resulted in a swelter of confusing claims and counterclaims of superiority; many proprietary systems purport to measure severity, but in fact measure nothing more than cost variation.

Decubitus ulcer constitutes an example of a comorbidity in which the severity of service may in fact be quite different from the severity of illness. In the APR-DRGs, a patient with a decubitus ulcer is placed into a class 3 (there are four classes in the APR-DRGs with class 1 being minor and class 4 termed extreme). There is likely to be no disagreement that a patient with a decubitus ulcer consumes more resources than a patient without one. But is that patient more severely ill simply by virtue of the fact that he or she has a decubitus ulcer? This is difficult to answer; clinical research is needed for a definitive response. Many clinicians would indicate that a pneumonia patient with a decubitus ulcer is not much more severely ill than one without. On the other hand, most clinicians would similarly agree that a diabetic patient with a decubitus ulcer is in fact more "severely" ill than one without such an ulcer. Thus while we might all agree that patients with decubitus ulcer represent a higher severity of service we do not clinically understand for many clinical situations whether these patients are, in fact, more severely ill. The many issues undergirding the above example demonstrate why there is confusion within both the academic research community and the marketplace about what the many competing severity of illness systems are actually measuring: severity of illness, severity of service, or both.

To compound the complexity of the severity issue, many clinicians as well as marketers of proprietary severity products encourage belief in the following hypothesis: increased severity of illness during a hospital stay (as measured by their system) correlates with increased problems in quality of care delivered to the patient. Little research has been performed to support this assertion. Recent research by Iezzoni et al. constitutes one of the few studies of this issue.[11] In this research, Iezzoni and her colleagues examined whether two frequently quoted severity of illness systems, CSI and Medisgrps, are able to identify quality of care problems. Worsening severity of illness for hospitalized patients was associated with physician assessments of quality problems. They found inconsistent correlation between increased severity and quality of care problems based on examination of the medical record. This inconsistency was particularly marked in Medisgrps, less so in CSI. In preliminary research, the author of this chapter examined one of the most common comorbidities—urinary tract infection (UTI). There was little correlation between increased severity of illness brought about by the presence of a UTI and poor quality of care.

Using the APR-DRGs in Your Clinical Practice

APR-DRGs represent the integration of the Yale DRG refinements with the AP-DRGs. APR-DRGs determine class assignments by examining the following aspects of a patient's stay in the hospital:

1. Each of the APR-DRGs is divided into four subclasses: minor, moderate, major, and extreme.
2. The APR-DRGs are based on AP-DRGs, not the HCFA DRGs. Thus, the base DRGs are relevant for the entire population as the HCFA DRGs are relevant for Medicare. For example, there are virtually no neonatal DRGs, a critically important fact for managed care organizations and physicians trying to manage these very expensive types of patients.

3. Class assignment is adjusted if the secondary diagnosis typically is part of the principal diagnosis. Thus, urinary retention, typically a class 2 type of comorbidity, becomes class 1 if the principal diagnosis is prostatic hypertrophy or if a transurethral resection of the prostate is performed.

4. Class assignment also is adjusted in the reverse direction. Thus an uncomplicated diabetic patient having a vaginal delivery is placed into a higher class by virtue of the diabetes itself.

5. Age, per se, constitutes a modifier. Thus, for example, pediatric patients with bone infections are placed into a higher class than adults with similar comorbidities. Bone infections in pediatric patients are frequently more severe due to the active growth plate in their bones.

6. The principal diagnosis itself may modify class assignment. Thus, for example, a patient with a principal diagnosis of diabetic hyperosmolar coma is certainly different from a straightforward diabetic patient—irrespective of any secondary diagnoses the two patients may have.

7. The performance of a non-operating room procedure, such as the im-plantation of a temporary pacemaker, can also sometimes serve to adjust the class assignment of a patient's comorbidities. Thus, for example, it is difficult, if not impossible, to assess the clinical significance of a patient with a complete heart block as a secondary diagnosis. It is certainly more than a class 1 secondary diagnosis; however, there is a range in the severity of illness of patients with a complete heart block. Some patients are walking around with this condition while others need immediate and intensive medical intervention. Thus, the class assignment of a patient with complete heart block is modified if a temporary pacemaker is implanted during the hospitalization.

8. The most significant theoretical advance in the APR-DRGs is that the interaction of secondary diagnosis is taken into account. This has represented a significant conundrum for researchers in the field. A thorough examination of the more severely ill patients is particularly important. For example, traditional DRG refinements have not been able to adequately

explain the severity of illness of patients in intensive care units. An examination of patients with multiple comorbid diagnoses represents a significant advance in the DRG refinement technology.

Multiple comorbidities are common among admitted patients. Thus a patient with out-of-control diabetes may have a pulmonary problem on top of congestive heart failure. Surely this patient is distinct from a diabetic patient with a decubitus ulcer and cellulitis. Not only are these patients clinically distinct but, more importantly, it is necessary to know whether these patients' multiple comorbidities interact. The APR-DRGs take into account the interaction of these multiple comorbidities.

From the following examples, managed care physicians will learn to:

1. utilize a case mix system developed for inpatient services
2. compare different hospitals looking at both cost and mortality
3. examine expected vs. actual data for charges, LOS, and mortality
4. appreciate the importance of working with medical staff and administrative leadership in a hospital in order to best understand sources of variation in resource consumption and quality of care.

An application of the revised and refined DRGs can be seen in the following example:

Case #1. Through the evaluation of one year's discharge data, 185,000 records were examined using the hospital system's expected average charges, LOS, and mortality on a comparative basis to evaluate each hospital's performance. The expected average relates to the average of charges, LOS, and mortality—which would have occured if the hospital's case mix by DRG by severity level had been treated at the hospital system's average. In several hospitals there were differences noted in charges, LOS, and mortality pertaining to several APR-DRGs.

Table 8–1 summarizes a report for one of the two DRGs, total cholecystectomy without common duct exploration. From Table 8–1, it would appear that patients falling into this DRG category at Hospital A cost more than the average for the Alternate Hospital System. Table 8–2 takes the DRG information provided in Table 8–1 and adjusts it to take into account the severity of the patients; it also summarizes the differences in charges between Hospital A and the Alternate Hospital System for DRG-197. Although the difference in average charge for this DRG is $1,101 higher at Hospital A than at the Alternate Hospital System, this calculation did not take into account the fact that patients who underwent cholecystectomy at Hospital A were sicker. If one statistically corrects for the fact that Hospital A's gallbladder-removal patients were sicker, the expected charge at Hospital A increases from $7,307 to $7,583. Therefore, Hospital A's costs for treated patients in DRG-197 are lower, rather than higher than expected, if nonseverity-adjusted DRGs are used.

There appears to be a clear difference between patients in this DRG at Hospital A and at the Alternate System. That is, within this DRG, patients in Hospital A are sicker than than those in the Alternate System, of which Hospital A is a part. Thus, patients at Hospital A who had a cholecystectomy also had more frequent secondary diagnoses.

Figure 8–1 provides the charges subdivided by severity class comparing Hospital A with the Alternate System. In this figure, one can see that adjustment by severity is the key to understanding why the charges at Hospital A are higher than those at the

---

Table 8–1 DRG 197 – Total Cholecystectomy without Common Duct Exploration

Hospital A Patients = 89   AHS Patients = 1,039

Average Charge Hospital A	7,307
Average Charge AHS	6,206
Charge Difference	-1,101
Expected Charge Hospital	7,583
Charge Difference	+276

Note: AHS–Alternate Hospital System

Source: 3M/HIS

Alternate System. Charges at Hospital A in severity class 1 are similar to those for the entire chain. In fact, in classes 3 and 4, after adjusting for severity, Hospital A's charges are less than those of the Alternate Hospital System.

Case #2. Table 8–3 provides important information on evaluating differences in mortality between hospitals within the Alternate Hospital System. That is, it appears that there may be a difference in mortality between patients hospitalized with pneumonia at Hospital A compared with the Alternate Hospital System. The difference is particularly obvious between class 1 and 2 patients; those patients who came to Hospital A with minor or moderate coexistent illnesses or complications had a higher mortality rate than patients who came to the Alternate Hospital System in a similar clinical condition. There is little difference in mortality between patients at Hospital A and patients at the Alternate Hospital System who are hospitalized with pneumonia and have severe complicating diseases such as myocardial infarction. This type of analysis can be helpful in guiding the course of quality management studies. It should be emphasized that results of APR-DRG investigations cannot be utilized as the final word on whether differences in mortality represent significant lapses in quality. They do indicate that further studies, typically onsite reviews or examinations of the medical records, are necessary.

The responses of both the medical staff and administrative leadership at Alternate Hospital System were noteworthy. On presentation of the data, impacted clinicians, administrators, and other members of the health care team worked together to change the

Table 8–2 DRG 197—Total Cholecystectomy without Common Duct Exploration

Severity	Hospital A Percentage	Charges	AHS Percentage	Charges	Charge Difference
1	30.3%	5,002	55.5%	5,011	+ 9
2	13.5%	5,789	24.8%	6,052	+ 263
3	48.3%	7,865	15.9%	8,129	+ 264
4	7.9%	15,371	3.8%	16,767	+1,396

Note: AHS, Alternate Hospital System.

Source: 3M/HIS.

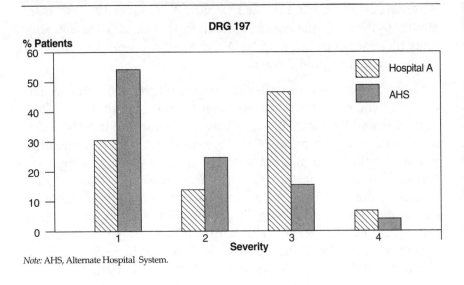

Note: AHS, Alternate Hospital System.

Figure 8–1 Summary of Differences in Charges. *Source:* 3M/HIS

care provided. This resulted in a reduction of the differences in mortality between Alternate Hospital System and Hospital A.*

The foregoing examples typify the type of work managed care physicians will be called on to perform in inpatient settings. Managed care companies have numerous hospitals under contract and will need to compare and contrast performance on a number of clinical variables over time. Once a severity adjustment tool is adopted by an institution, a managed care physician might adopt the following strategy for implementation: If there is top leadership support for quality improvement and a belief in the value of severity-adjusted case mix data, then over a period of time, comparisons between classes of patients should be performed. Examination of data over time should then be plotted on a graph utilizing a control chart methodology, thus identifying whether or not a difference in—for example—cost represents a true difference or a random event. If the differences do remain, comparison of groups of patients in similar classes will reveal whether or not these classes of patients contain differences in costs. If so, it would not be unreasonable to ask why such a differ-

*Information drawn from 3M/HIS

Table 8–3 Mortality Differences within the Alternate Hospital System

Hospital A
DRG 89 Simple Pneumonia Age>17

Severity	Patients	Hospital Mortality	AHS Mortality	Severity
1	77	5.2%	1.0%	- 4.2%
2	93	9.7%	3.9%	- 5.8%
3	23	17.4%	16.7%	- 0.7%

Note: AHS, Alternate Hospital System.

Source: 3M/HIS

ence exists. If the methodology defining the severity of illness classes is valid, two possiblities exist: either the cost differentials between the two groups of patients in the same class represent differences in practice style that resulted in unnecessary utilization of services or problems in quality resulted from the increased utilization of services to rectify the quality of care problems.

If administrative leadership is neither supportive nor clear on the benefits of case mix systems, the managed care physician must work with the medical director and create strong physician understanding of and support for the case mix system. Clinically reasonable and claims-based inpatient case mix systems represent an important advance in our efforts to understand the sources of variation in resource consumption and quality of care.

RECENT TRENDS IN APG AND DRG DEVELOPMENT

Several development efforts pertaining to DRGs and APGs are currently underway:

1. APR-DRGs are continually being refined, with emphasis on understanding specific aspects of interactions between co-morbidities and primary/secondary diagnoses. Current research will likely improve the capacity of these case mix systems to measure variance of cost, LOS, or other variables.

2. At a more clinically interesting level, continued research on large administrative databases will provide clinical information on the reasons a particular comorbidity or complication

consumes significant resources. Thus, the high cost of UTIs, applicable to all classes of patients regardless of age or sex, constitutes a specific and common comorbidity. However, there is little understanding of the clinical reasons for the expensive comorbidity of UTIs.

3. Significant research studies will be conducted in an effort to better understand the different uses of hospital case mix systems within the quality improvement process. For example, the research group at 3M/HIS is currently testing APR-DRGs at a large teaching hospital in the northeastern United States to determine how they are utilized over a period of two years. Specific interventions, developed after an examination of APR-DRG data, will be examined. The medical community is just beginning to understand the most effective management strategies for integrating DRG refinement data into the quality improvement process.

4. A significant amount of refinement is ongoing in the Medical APGs. Current research is examining the value of including patient health status information in APG construction. Under particular examination is this hypothesis: Does the combination of the diagnosis and health status of the patient improve the ability of the medical APG to predict resource consumption?

5. With ongoing refinement of APGs and APR-DRGs, questions have already arisen regarding the use of these case mix systems in the development of episodes of care.

6. National health reform may attempt to balance regulatory with market-based approaches to health care delivery. Recent writing has documented how DRGs and APGs could fit into such a strategy.[12] It is likely that experiments utilizing prospective payment in conjunction with procompetitive market-based approaches will be attempted over the next few years.

7. In the past several years, international interest in case mix applications has exploded. Rising health care costs, in combination with a downturn in many world industrial economies, have prompted renewed commitment to understanding costs of health care operations. The long and successful track record of DRGs has led policymakers to focus on this approach. Portuguese physicians and health care managers recently developed their own Portuguese National DRGs that,

beginning in 1992, were implemented in a fashion analogous to our Medicare system.* In Sweden, where health services are managed at the county level, many counties are using either AP-DRGs or HCFA DRGs for hospital budgeting purposes. Many other countries are looking at DRGs and their variants in examining health care costs of their hospitals.

CONCLUSION

This chapter has attempted to provide the managed care physician with an understanding of

1. the most commonly utilized case mix systems for inpatient and outpatient services
2. how these systems can be used to understand the sources of variation in resource consumption and aspects of quality of care
3. the utility of these systems for contracting purposes
4. the use of these systems as a communications tool between physicians working within the same institution to improve care and lower cost.

As managed care continues to proliferate, case mix systems will better enable us to understand issues pertaining to cost and quality. Depending on their role in the public or private sector, policymakers throughout the world are increasingly making use of the inpatient and outpatient case mix measures described herein. New York State has already adopted the New York APGs. It is likely that the federal government will adopt one or more of these measures as payment for ambulatory services. On the inpatient side, DRGs are already established in the United States. Our health care future also portends the increased use of refined DRGs, particularly in the quality improvement process.

Decision makers in the private sector will also make increased use of the inpatient and ambulatory measures discussed herein. This is particularly true on the managed care side, whether the provider is paid on a capitated (per patient per month) or discounted fee-for-service basis. As described from both a theoretical

---

*Communication from J. Vertress, Solon Consulting, Bethesda, MD.

and case history perspective, physicians working in managed care organizations will want to utilize case mix systems that, from a clinical and resource consumption perspective, accurately describe the basic building blocks of inpatient and outpatient services.

For the true believers in the quality improvement movement, it is arguable whether we should pay attention to outcomes of care, rather than case mix systems. On the surface, case mix systems bear no relation to outcomes. Many hospital-based providers view case mix systems such as DRGs as Medicare's "draconian noose" (in the form of inadequate payment). This chapter forcefully demonstrates that the applicability of case mix systems extends far beyond payment purposes; it also serves as a means of measuring outcomes (analyses of morbidity and mortality) and processes.

Finally, an effective quality improvement program must include adequate institutional support for the CQI process. Critical to improvement of the process is a thorough institutional commitment to understanding the information through tools that help describe both processes and outcomes of care. Case mix tools represent a critical element in that armory.

REFERENCES

1. Russell L. *Medicare's New Hospital Payment System*. Washington, DC: The Brookings Institution; 1989.

2. Leader S, Moon M. Medicare trends in ambulatory surgery. *Health Affairs*. Spring 1989.

3. Averill R, Goldfield N, McGuire T, et al. Design and development of a prospective payment system for ambulatory care. Final report. Prepared with the support of the Health Care Financing Administration; December 1990.

4. Codman EA. The product of a hospital. *Surgery, Gynecology, and Obstetrics*. 1914;18:491–496.

5. Fetter RB, Brand DA, Gamache D. DRGs: their design and development. Ann Arbor, MI: *Health Administration Press*; 1991:4,12.

6. Schwartz W, Mendelson D. Hospital cost containment in the 1980's—hard lessons learned and prospects for the 1990s. *N Engl J Med*. 1991;234(15):1037–1042.

7. Davis K, Anderson GE, Rowland D, Steinberg E. *Health Care Cost Containment*. Baltimore, MD: Johns Hopkins University Press; 1990:173.

8. Nelson EC, Berwick DM. The measurement of health status in clincial practice. *Medical Care*. 1989;27(3):577–590.

9. Barksy AJ III. Hidden reasons some patients visit doctors. *Ann Inter Med*. 1981;94:492.

10. Burnum J. The worried sick. *Ann Inter Med*. 1978;88:572.

11. Iezzoni LI, Ash AS, Coffman GA, Moskowitz MA. Predicting in-hospital mortality. *Medical Care*. 1992;30(4):347–359.

12. Averill R, Kalison M. Competition and prospective payment: a new way to control health care costs. *J Am Health Policy*. March/April 1993:22–28.

Editorial Commentary

Susan L. Howell
David B. Nash

Physicians will be increasingly responsible for learning new tools that enhance understanding of both resource consumption and quality assurance. Among these tools are case mix, or clinical classification systems—bundles of care treatments for clinically coherent groups of patients. Diagnosis-Related Groups (DRGs), developed by HCFA as a means of Medicare prospective inpatient reimbursement, are perhaps the best known type of case mix system.

The trend toward outpatient care has resulted in the fairly recent development of ambulatory case mix systems such as Ambulatory patient groups (APGs). Like DRGs, ambulatory case mix systems are becoming increasingly sophisticated and used not only as a payment mechanism but as a means of utilization management and quality improvement. Ambulatory case mix systems hold particular promise for managed care organizations because of managed care's emphasis on preventive and outpatient treatment.

Dr. Norbert Goldfield draws upon his experience as a medical director at the CIGNA and 3M/HIS Corporation for this chapter. The 3M/HIS Corporation is currently under contract with the HCFA to develop APGs, and is considered one of the international leaders in this area. Dr. Goldfield leads us into what for many was unknown territory. This chapter aims to provide an introduction to case mix systems without being overly technical. For those with a more advanced knowledge, Dr. Goldfield's "cutting edge" vantage point is sure to offer new information and insights into this rapidly evolving field.

Dr. Goldfield describes the latest developments in inpatient and outpatient case mix systems, including severity-adjusted DRGs, and their respective components and applications for medical care review. He also explains the difficulties inherent in classifying the ambulatory encounter and how this has posed challenges in the development of ambulatory case mix systems (ACMS). As Dr. Goldfield emphasizes, ACMS may well be the long-awaited missing link—in the guise of an economic "knot"—that can tie physicians and hospitals together.

Case mix systems in general, Dr. Goldfield asserts, can provide a wealth of information about the process and outcome of care. However, he cautions that institutional support and a commitment to understanding the information provided by case mix systems are imperative if they are to be truly effective.

Chapter 9

Managed Care: Its Relationship with Organized Medicine and Its Role in Future Health Care Policy Proposals

Kenneth R. Epstein

INTRODUCTION

Medical science has undergone many changes over the past century. The development of antibiotics, the discovery of the role of insulin in diabetes mellitus, and the development of coronary artery bypass surgery are but a few examples. Paralleling these changes in the science of medicine are the continued changes in the organization and financing of health care in the United States. In the late 19th and early 20th centuries, solo practice was by far the predominant arrangement for practicing medicine.[1] Over the course of the 20th century, the types of practice arrangements have grown to include not only solo practice but small partnerships, large group practices, salaried positions with hospitals and other health care organizations, and many others. Managed care has grown as well, from just a theoretical concept less than 20 years ago, to a central component of many present-day health insurance organizations. With the looming specter of out-of-control health care costs and increasing numbers of Americans lacking health insurance, the practice environment will change even more in the years ahead.

Physicians in general, and organized medicine in particular, have attempted to respond to these changes in ways that reflected concern for both quality of health care and the economic security of individual practitioners. During this period, the American Medical Association (AMA) has grown from an organization of only 8,000 physicians at the turn of the century to a huge organization of several hundred thousand members that represents close to 50 percent of all practicing physicians.[1] Understanding the changes in the AMA's position on health care issues thus provides a means of understanding the changes in the profession in general. The future configuration of the health care system depends in part on the attitudes of the AMA and other medical organizations toward various proposed changes.

This chapter serves two purposes. The first is to examine the changes in organized medicine's attitudes toward managed care over the past 20 years. Managed care organizations have grown rapidly, from experimental models involving few patients to one of the predominant types of health care insurance structures in this country. Organized medicine's response to these changes has reflected their perceptions of who their members are and what they want.

The second goal of this chapter is to examine in detail the various proposals—currently under discussion nationally—to reform the American health care system. Clearly, managed care will play an important role in all of the health care proposals, but the specifics of how central the role will be differs significantly among them. Knowing the specifics of the various proposals and how managed care would fit in can aid in understanding the advantages and disadvantages of various forms of health care reform.

MANAGED CARE: THE PROFESSION'S INITIAL REACTION

Support of the concept of prepaid group practice has existed since the 1920s.[2] However, due in large part to the AMA's known opposition, there were few attempts to incorporate these concepts into public policy. In the 1950s, prepaid group practice was again actively discussed. Again the AMA strongly opposed the concept.[3] This opposition was well known, and prevented government from seriously promoting its growth.[2]

The 1970s: Nixon Administration Advocacy

In the early 1970s, the HMO concept began to be discussed in earnest. Two events prompted this reevaluation. The first was the publication of Paul Ellwood's article that described in detail the theoretical advantage of HMOs.[4] He argued that a "health maintenance industry" was necessary to counter an increase in government intervention and regulation. This industry would be based on the creation of HMOs that could provide more economical and effective services than conventional fee-for-service providers.

With the publication of Ellwood's article, there was a simultaneous increase in pressure on the Nixon administration to devise a health care proposal that could deal with the increasing cost of health care. The administration made Ellwood's HMO concept the centerpiece of their plans. Since they would be run by private industry, HMOs obviated the need for government involvement. They were thus quite attractive to the Republican administration.[5] Nixon proposed the creation, by 1976, of 1,700 HMOs, with an enrollment of 40 million people. His goal was to make HMOs available to 90 percent of the population by 1980.[1] With the onset of the Watergate scandal, however, the Nixon administration's initiative collapsed. A severe economic recession further eroded interest in health care program development.[1]

Again, in the 1920s and 1950s, organized medicine—specifically the AMA—strongly opposed the growth of HMOs. The patient population eligible for enrollment in HMOs consisted of those currently obtaining health care through the fee-for-service system. The growth of HMOs thus directly threatened the economic interests of private practitioners. Consequently, the AMA, who represented these private practitioners, vehemently opposed any federal legislation that would encourage HMO growth.[6]

The combination of the loss of the Nixon administration's advocacy and the strong opposition by the AMA slowed the growth of HMOs in the 1970s.[1] However, Congress did pass several bills that assisted the development of HMOs. In 1976, Congress reduced federal requirements that limited HMO growth. Then, in 1978, federal aid to HMOs was increased. As a result, by 1979 there were only 217 HMOs with 7.9 million persons enrolled, far short of Nixon's original plan.[1]

The 1980s and 1990s: The Changing Balance between Managed Care and Fee-for-Service

Significant changes occurred in the health care landscape during the 1980s. For example, in response to societal pressure to control Medicare spending, the Reagan administration, in 1983, passed legislation that authorized standardized inpatient-care payment by diagnosis-related groups.[3] During the decade, the number of HMOs more than tripled.[7] Likewise, the number of HMO enrollees skyrocketed, from only 6 million in 1976 to over 38 million by 1991.[8] In 1987, 41 percent of health insurance policies were still conventional indemnity insurance without explicit utilization management, as opposed to 27 percent of policies being HMOs or preferred provider organizations (PPOs).[9] By 1991, only 5 percent of health insurance policies remained conventional indemnity without utilization management, whereas the percentage of HMO- or PPO-based policies had risen to 43 percent.[9] It is estimated that presently, over 50 percent of physicians have at least one HMO contract.[8, 10]

These changes are affecting all specialties. For example, more and more psychiatrists are joining managed care systems.[11] Likewise, opportunities for managed care employment for internists have become prevalent enough that in many communities, managed care organizations can now dictate internists' salary ranges.[12]

Practitioners nationwide, from the heart of Appalachia to the largest coastal cities, have been affected by the changing health care landscape. Physicians in small towns and rural areas are increasingly accepting the role of managed care insurance systems in their communities.[13] Likewise, in major metropolitan areas, physicians are noting an increasing number of employers purchasing health care for their employees through HMOs.[14] Therefore, many physicians join independent practice associations in order to compete for HMO contracts.

Organized medicine's attitude toward managed health care has reflected the many changes in health care financing that have occurred over the past ten years. Aware of the demographic changes in physician practices, it has attempted to adjust accordingly. As recently as 1990, most articles in the *Journal of the*

American Medical Association (JAMA) and the *American Medical News* continued to predominantly portray the perceived negatives of managed care. The main criticisms concerned loss of patients' ability to freely choose providers and loss of physicans' ability to set their own rates. A 1990 *JAMA* article by the Office of the General Counsel of the AMA explained how large health care payers maintain unfair control over the market.[15]

Since late 1992, the AMA has taken a more neutral stance. Robert E. McAffee, MD, and vice-chairman of the AMA Board of Trustees, has said that the AMA does not explicitly oppose managed care.[16] However, he also confirmed that the AMA does believe that patients' needs are better served by free-market competition and free choice among physicians and patients. The American College of Physicians (ACP) has actively supported the increasing role of managed care in America. During the ACP's annual meeting in 1992, panel discussions were conducted on the pros and cons of managed care vs. fee-for-service.[17] In the fall of 1992, the ACP proposed major changes in the health care system that would give managed care a central role.[18] This is discussed in more detail later in the chapter.

Organized medicine's attitude toward large group practices and the growth of managed care does not simply reflect economic philosophy. The AMA and other medical organizations have come to realize that significantly fewer of their real or potential members fit the mold of the fee-for-service solo practitioner. In 1965, only 11 percent of nonfederal physicians practiced in groups, but by 1991, that number increased to 36 percent.[10] Organized medicine therefore now realizes that it needs these physicians as members. Dr. James Todd, AMA executive vice-president, at the 1992 meeting of the Group Health Association of America (GHAA), publicly stated for the first time that the AMA "accepted the legitimacy and the benefits of [HMOs]."[10] In response to Dr. Todd's statement, GHAA President James Doherty asserted that physicians practicing HMO medicine would now be willing to join the AMA. The sensitivity of this very political issue quickly prompted representatives of private practice medicine to criticize Dr. Todd's overtures to the managed care industry. They threatened that long-time AMA members would quit "by the thousands" in protest.[10]

However, with greater numbers of physicians practicing in these settings, the AMA has come to realize that managed care physicians also must be welcomed to their organization. "If the AMA is going to represent all doctors . . . you can't take the doctors who practice in groups and ignore them. They need representation, too."[10]

THE FUTURE OF MANAGED CARE: ITS ROLE IN HEALTH CARE REFORM

The AMA, and organized medicine in general, has attempted to respond to the recent changes in the health care system and to stay in line with the demographics of its membership. No one knows what the future will hold for U.S. health care in the 1990s. Proposals have been discussed that deal with the dual problems of increasing health care costs and lack of access to health care. Some proposals advocate a fine-tuning of the present system, and others recommend a radical reshaping of the entire system.

No matter what form the future health care system takes, it is clear that managed care is here to stay. Managed care may occur only within part of the system, as is presently true, or the future system may be designed around the concepts of managed care. In either case, there will be a major change in outlook toward managed care physicians. Increasingly, managed care physicians will become the standard against which traditional fee-for-service physicians will be judged. Therefore, it is crucial that managed care physicians understand their central role in the future of health care, regardless of the eventual form of the system. Only time will tell if the future health care system in the United States will resemble one of these proposals, or will be a combination of parts of all of them.

The following discussion centers on the key health care proposals currently being considered—proposals with an emphasis on the role of managed care.

GOVERNMENT PROPOSALS

Pepper Commission Report

The United States Bipartisan Commission on Comprehensive Health Care was created by Congress in the late 1980s to recommend legislative action ensuring coverage for health and long-term care for all Americans. The commission was named the Pepper Commission in honor of the late Senator Claude Pepper of Florida. It unanimously concluded that the need for federal action was urgent, but that any changes should build on and strengthen the present combination of job-based and public coverage.[19] Despite agreement on these general principles, the commission was unable to agree on the details of their proposed program. Therefore, the specific recommendations passed by a vote of 8 to 7, largely along partisan lines.

The Pepper Commission recommendations are based on two themes: building universal coverage and strengthening the present health care system. As previously noted, the commission recommended ensuring universal coverage through refinement of the present system of both employer-based and public health insurance plans. Large employers would be required to provide coverage for their employees. Small employers would be encouraged through tax credits and subsidies to provide health insurance coverage for their employees. The federal government would provide coverage for the unemployed and the poor by replacing and expanding the present state-run Medicaid programs.

The Pepper Commission discussed the role of government, employers, and individuals in sharing the cost of financing this expanded health insurance coverage. Both private insurers and the government would be involved in administering these programs.

The second key element of the Pepper Commission report involved efforts to strengthen the health care system. The commission asserted that the country needs a national quality assurance system aimed at defining appropriate or necessary services and ensuring that patients have access to these services. It recommended the development and implementation of national practice guidelines as standards of care. It also argued for the establishment of a minimum benefit package that, except for preventive services, involves significant consumer cost sharing.

The Pepper Commission's report specifically advocates managed care as an appropriate means of service delivery for employers as well as the federal government. The commission's recommendations for insurance system reform would further encourage managed care and other cost management innovations. They argue that competition within the health care system should be based on efficient service and management of health care expenditures.

Health USA

The Health USA Act was introduced to the United States Senate in 1991 by Senator Bob Kerrey of Nebraska.[20] This proposal aims to provide universal health insurance coverage through a joint federal-state program funded through taxes, rather than the present system of premium-funded private insurance. The proposal is based on individual state administration of health insurance programs, with the federal government providing guidelines and financial support. All state residents would be covered by the state health insurance system. However, service would be obtained by enrollment in one of the local private health plans, such as competing fee-for-service plans, HMOs, and other existing plans. If no local plans were available, or if a resident preferred, he or she could enroll in a state-run plan.

By recommending that the state program pay individual health plans for the provision of service, the Health USA proposal strongly emphasizes managed care and prepaid health plans as the predominant model of care. The state program would make a capitation payment to each plan covering all enrollees. The plan must then provide all federally mandated benefits to the enrolled member. By emphasizing capitated payment to competing health care plans, the Health USA proposal places increased emphasis on primary care. The primary care provider would have a central role in most local plans. The provision of preventive health care services would be mandated by the federal government. However, providing preventive care would also be in the best interests of the local health care plan: in a capitated system, it is advantageous to the plan to keep its enrollees healthy.

As in several of the other proposals, a central provision of the Health USA proposal is the separation of health insurance from employment.[20] Individuals and families could choose any approved plan available in their area, rather than choosing from the few plans offered by their employer. By untying coverage from employment, an individual would not risk changing plans and physicians when changing jobs, or if faced with unemployment or disability. Likewise, there would be no changes in physician or plan necessitated by divorce from a covered spouse or retirement from work.

The Health USA proposal differs in several respects from other proposals.[20] Like Enthoven'and Kronick's "consumer-choice" plan discussed later in the section "A 'Consumer-Choice' Model," this proposal strongly emphasizes prepaid health plans.[21] The Enthoven and Kronick proposal relies on market forces to increase cost-consciousness among individual payers and health care providers. Competi-tion between providers will control costs. The Health USA proposal, by contrast, advocates the creation of a unified all-payer reimbursement system as a necessary step in changing the financial incentives to health plans and providers and promoting cost-efficient health care.

The Health USA proposal differs from other single payer systems such as the Canadian health care system or the Physicians for a National Health Program (PNHP).[22] These systems preserve private practice fee-for-service medicine as the predominant model of health care delivery. The proponents of the Health USA proposal argue that this insulates practitioners from efforts to improve the cost-effectiveness of health care expenditures.[20] The Health USA proposal, by contrast, mandates that state payment to health care plans be made in a capitated, prepaid mechanism, thereby encouraging an efficient, primary care-based system. The proponents of the Health USA proposal might argue that their proposal combines the administrative efficiency of the PNHP with the economic efficiency of managed care as proposed by Enthoven and Kronick.

A SINGLE-PAYER SYSTEM: THE PNHP

In 1989, the PNHP published its proposal for reforming the American health care system.[22] In contrast to several other proposals, most notably the AMA's "Health Access America,"[23] the PNHP proposal is based on the premise that the present U.S. health care system is failing. It therefore recommends fundamental changes in the system, namely the development of a comprehensive national health program.

The essence of the PNHP proposal is that all Americans would be covered by a single publicly financed and administered health insurance plan. Although the system would be federally mandated and funded, it could be administered at the state and local level. Funding for this publicly run program would be obtained through a combination of several sources. These sources would include funds from the current Medicare and Medicaid programs; the monies that employers currently pay for health care benefits; private health insurance company revenues; and, if necessary, additional revenues from increases in income taxes.

All services judged to be medically necessary would be included. Boards of experts and community representatives would be created in order to determine which services to include or exclude from coverage. As part of this universal single-payer coverage, all deductibles and copayments would be eliminated. The PNHP's justification for a single comprehensive system is that this is the only way to ensure equal access to care. The PHNP additionally argues that this system is necessary to reduce the complexity and expense of billing and administration inherent in the present system, with its myriad of private and public payers.

Physicians could be paid by one of three methods in the single-payer system:

1. Fee-for-service would be continued for physicians currently practicing under this method of payment. A simplified, binding fee schedule would be created by a state national health program payment board that would include representatives from the fee-for-service practitioners. Since payment would be only through the single national health program,

billing would be simplified, and could be done electronically. Physicians could directly bill patients for uncovered services only.
2. Physicians employed by institutions such as hospitals and health centers could be paid by salary. These institutions would in turn be paid by a global budget that would cover all operating expenses, rather than billing for services provided.
3. Organizations such as HMOs, group practices, or other similar settings could be paid by capitation, again with the rates set to cover all operating expenses. Physicians practicing in these settings would be salaried. The present diversity of existing practice arrangements would therefore be preserved.

The PNHP proposal does not address whether there would be any change in the role of managed care in their health care system. HMOs and other current managed care programs could be maintained. Likewise, the PNHP's proposal would not discourage the perpetuation of fee-for-service payments to practitoners. However, managed care would likely have a prominent role for a different reason: Since the universal health insurance system would be publicly financed and administered, and additional health care spending could be financed only through higher taxes, there would be incredible public pressure on the system to control costs and spend efficiently. Therefore, both federal and state administrators would likely implement methods of efficient health care resource management. These methods would probably involve control of the primary care/specialty mix of the medical profession as well as patient referral for specialty care and procedures.

Additionally, by changing to an annual lump-sum payment system to cover their "global budget," all providers would be under added pressure to manage resources efficiently. Large capital expenditures could not come out of this global budget, but would be funded separately. Therefore, there would be additional pressure to justify capital expenditures. If large purchases, such as a magnetic resonance imaging (MRI) scanner or additional hospital beds could not be justified in terms of community needs, then they most likely would not be financed. This community needs assessment prior to capital expenditures further exemplifies the essential role that managed care would play in the PNHP's health care system.

A "CONSUMER-CHOICE" MODEL: ENTHOVEN'S AND KRONICK'S PROPOSAL

Concurrent with the 1989 publication of the PNHP proposal, Alain Enthoven and Richard Kronick of Stanford University published their health plan.[21] Their model is the most explicit in that it recommends the United States move toward managed care health insurance systems as the predominant health care payment method of the future. They argue that in the current, predominantly fee-for-service system there is no incentive to practice medicine in an efficient, cost-effective manner. By contrast, managed care systems such as HMOs and PPOs have the potential to create serious cost-consciousness among providers and patients.

As do proponents of many of the other proposals, Enthoven and Kronick argue for comprehensive change in the American health care delivery system. They assert that attempts to control costs through cost-conscious use of managed care will not be successful if elsewhere in the system, open-ended demand is driving up prices and standards of care. They ask, "Why should doctors and hospitals accept serious cost containment by HMOs if there is plenty of open-minded demand for their services elsewhere?"[21] The inefficiency of the system—by eating up resources—promotes problems of access to care. Therefore, Enthoven and Kronick believe that a satisfactory strategy for health care delivery must simultaneously tackle the inefficient excesses in the system and the problems of deficient access to care.

In Enthoven's and Kronick's model, all Americans would be covered by health insurance, either through their employers, or through the development of "public sponsor" agencies. These agencies would be based on federal legislation that would support the development of public sponsors, or insurance brokers, at the state level. These public sponsors would select the coverages to be offered, contract with health plans and beneficiaries about rules of participation, manage the enrollment process, collect premium contributions from beneficiaries, pay premiums to health plans, and administer both cross-subsidies among beneficiaries and subsidies available to the whole group.[21] They could contract with many different managed care plans, as many large employers are presently doing.

Enthoven and Kronick argue that a free market insurance system will not result in an efficient or fair health care system. Strategies such as market segmentation, refusals to insure certain high-risk persons, and excluding pre-existing systems are some of the ways in which a health insurance system left to market forces would inhibit universal health insurance coverage. Enthoven and Kronick therefore argue for a system they call "managed competition," in which the public sponsors could contract with competing health plans to ensure cost-conscious, informed consumer choice.[21]

Enthoven's and Kronick's proposal would encourage the growth of efficient managed care organizations. As with health maintenance organizations, the functions of insurance and provision of care would probably be integrated into most plans. A variety of systems and oganizations could still exist, with those that provide the best, most efficient health care coverage having a competitive advantage in attracting the public sponsors' business. Although traditional fee-for-service practitioners would be allowed in this system, they would have an enormous disadvantage in attracting public sponsorship, given their inherent economic inefficiency. Physicians would gradually shift their locus of activity away from fee-for-service to managed care organizations. Just as the plans would compete for contractual relationships with the public and employer sponsors, these managed care companies would also compete for the best physicians, and would attempt to promote physician loyalty. The organizations that treated their physicians the best would, in theory, have the happiest, most efficient health care providers, who in turn would provide the best care for the price. These companies would therefore be able to acquire more contracts with public sponsors, which in turn would enable them to pay the physicians more and encourage maximum physician loyalty. This would start the cycle over again.

In summary, Enthoven's and Kronick's proposed system is one in which all Americans would be covered by health insurance, through either their employer or a public sponsor. The insurance companies would compete for contracts with the sponsors. This competition would spur the growth of managed care institutions, based on cost-efficiency and quality. Enthoven and Kronick envision that within several years, economic forces will lead all health insurance systems toward prepaid, managed care.

PROPOSALS BY ORGANIZED MEDICINE

The AMA Plan: "Health Access America"

In February 1990, the AMA published a proposal calling for change within the health care system in order to improve access and control costs.[23] The plan was termed "Health Access America." Unlike other proposals, a key tenet of the AMA's premise is that the American health care system is fundamentally sound, and therefore does not require major changes. In the background section of its proposal, the AMA stresses the outstanding level of health care in the United States, and the high degree of patient satisfaction with the quality of medical care.[23] In defense of the present system, the AMA states that the cornerstones are patients' freedom of choice and a free and independent medical profession.[23]

In order to ensure access to care for all Americans, the AMA proposes three specific changes:

1. Major reforms in the Medicaid system would be required to provide uniform benefits to all persons below the poverty level. These benefits must be mandated to ensure equal benefits regardless of the state in which the individual resides.
2. Employers must provide health insurance to all their employees. Small and new businesses would be assisted through the creation of tax incentives and risk pools.
3. For those deemed the medically uninsurable and those unable to obtain coverage through Medicaid, Medicare, or their employer, state-level risk pools would be created in all states.

In order to ensure access for the elderly, the AMA advocates reform of the Medicare system. They also propose long-term coverage, funded through either the private insurance market or Medicaid.

The Health Access America proposal also considers means to reduce the high cost of health care. Several changes are recommended. The first is professional liability reform, the argument being that the practice of defensive medicine is driving up health care costs. Also proposed is the development of professional practice parameters. This would include establishing new recommendations for patient care, as well as maintaining accepted standards of care. Other recommendations for lowering health care costs include reducing incentives to overinsure through tax incentives, educating patients about cost-conscious health care, and encouraging health promotion and disease prevention.

A strong principle of the AMA plan is that patients must remain free to choose their physician and health care delivery system. The Health Access America proposal allows for the existence of managed care systems, as long as patient enrollment is voluntary. Although not explicitly stated, the AMA would oppose any effort to move the entire health care system toward managed care, as Enthoven and Kronick (as well as others) might propose.[21] The plan also recommends efforts to reduce the administrative costs of health care delivery by decreasing the "excessive and complicated paperwork nightmare" faced by patients and physicians.[23] The AMA also states, "The frustration of physicians in dealing with differing managed care requirements of multiple insurance companies . . . results in increased costs and interference with the physician-patient relationship."[23]

The proposal therefore addresses managed care in the context of criticism of the various requirements, both private and governmental, imposed upon the many insurance companies. Not addressed are the theoretical advantages or disadvantages of insurance companies utilizing managed care approaches in the first place. Several aspects of managed care are considered, but the AMA neither encourages nor condemns the growth of these systems. As previously noted, the AMA believes that selection of a health insurance plan should be based on voluntary choice. This is in contrast to proposals that advocate a fundamental shift toward managed care as the predominant system. In the context of reducing the administrative burden for physicians and their patients, the AMA also strongly argues against individual insurance companies' determining their own method of controlling costs through managed care approaches. The AMA proposal just as vehemently argues for preserving physicans' freedom to practice in the setting of their choice. It strongly opposes any system that would push physicians toward managed care organizations and remove their option of private practice. In Health Access America, a move toward managed care is clearly not viewed as an important or necessary goal of a reformed health care system.

The American College of Physicians Proposal

In September 1992, the ACP presented its proposal for the reformation of the American health care system.[18] Its argument was that universal access can be achieved only through systemwide change in the organization and financing of health care. The proposal, published in the *Annals of Internal Medicine*, described three aspects of the health care system it considers particularly troubling: (1) the present system promotes inequity and conflict between its private and public components, (2) benefit packages are based more on the needs of the payers than those of the patients, and (3) cost-control efforts have failed to make the system affordable and have resulted in an ever-increasing bureaucratic hassle for both physicians and patients.

The ACP suggests that these problems are remediable through fundamental reform of the health care system. It proposes the creation of a system of universal health insurance that would cover all U.S. citizens. The ACP envisions a pluralistic system that preserves the current variety of practice arrangements, which range from traditional fee-for-service to various organized managed care delivery systems. Universal access would be ensured by covering all Americans under either employer-sponsored or publicly sponsored insurance plans. Additionally, covered benefits would be mandated, and therefore would be the same for everyone. These benefits would be determined by a national health care commission, ensuring that all medically effective and appropriate services are covered. The health care commission would include representation from patients, physicians, other health care professionals, employers, insurers, government, and other key sectors of society.

As stated earlier, all individuals would be covered under either employer-financed or publicly financed health insurance. Theoretically, patients and providers would perceive no difference in health care between the employer-sponsored and publicly sponsored plans since only the source of financing would be different. Employers must either provide health insurance for their employees or pay an increased tax to help support the cost of the employees' coverage under the public system. The ACP proposes various means of making health insurance affordable to employers and encouraging employers to offer health insurance rather than pay out to public programs.

The ACP asserts that an insurance-based system would best allow for a wide range of practice arrangements that would suit the needs and preferences of patients and providers.[18] All insurance companies would offer, by mandate, the same benefit package, and payment rates for all payers would be uniform. Therefore, companies would have to compete on the basis of other characteristics, such as improved administrative efficiency or extra service at a slightly higher price.

Perhaps the most controversial component of the ACP's proposal is its recommendation that a national health care budget, or "global budget," be established. This would serve the purpose of setting a ceiling on expenditures, and encourage the health care system to manage resources efficiently. One possible method of controlling costs is to encourage increased reliance on managed care health insurance plans (in addition to negotiating prices with fee-for-service practitioners) based on a systematic, research-based method of valuing services. In addition to managing price, the ACP also recommends managing supply through the use of regulatory approaches. Demand would be controlled through patient education, simplifying the claims process.

In summary, the ACP proposal suggests maintaining the present types of health insurance, such as fee-for-service, HMOs, and PPOs. However, it advocates creating a global national budget for health care to put pressure on the health care system to manage resources efficiently. This would inevitably lead to the growth of managed care methods of health insurance, since an unmanaged fee-for-service system would cause a progressive increase in health care spending. Both employers and public payers would feel the financial pressure, leading both to most likely favor managed care systems.

The American Society of Internal Medicine Proposal

The American Society of Internal Medicine (ASIM) has proposed a system for health care reform entitled *Ending Separate and Unequal Health Care*.[24] The ASIM proposal seeks to maintain the existing health care financing system with its private health insurers as well as public programs such as Medicare and Medicaid. As with the other proposals, its goals are to ensure universal access to health insurance for all Americans, and improve the efficiency and cost-effectiveness of health care.

The ASIM is a national organization of internists and internal medicine subspecialists. Its goal is to impact the socioeconomic and political arenas of health care in order to protect the interests of its members and its patients. The majority of ASIM's members are private practitioners involved in the fee-for-service health insurance system. ASIM's health policy recommendations, therefore, seek to solve the problems of access to care and rising costs without negatively impacting the future of members who are involved in the fee-for-service system.

The ASIM proposal strongly supports the concept of employment-linked health insurance as the basis of any proposed changes in health care financing. The proposal states that " . . . most businesses . . . do a good job of offering health insurance to their employees. The most effective national strategy would be directed toward the minority of businesses that currently do not offer health insurance.[24] It further states that "Improvements in the current-employer-based system—rather than a complete shift away from job-based insurance—makes sense." The ASIM also recommends restructuring Medicaid away from a "welfare" program toward one that provides health insurance coverage for any person—regardless of income—who cannot obtain insurance through his or her employer.

The ASIM proposal argues forcibly against the concept of a single-payer health care system. It maintains that a single-payer system would result in insufficient access to medical technology, hospital beds, and elective surgery. The system, according to the ASIM proposal, would eliminate choices for patients and employers. The ASIM also believes that claims of administrative savings are greatly exaggerated. The proposal is therefore founded on the preservation of the existing multiple-payer system.

The ASIM proposal makes no specific mention of managed care's role in the future of health care. To the extent that it would not adversely affect ASIM members in private practice, the proposal would support managed care as part of a pluralistic free market health care system. However, the proposal's statement that a single-payer health care system would eliminate choices for patients and employers implies that the ASIM would oppose any health care model that supports government intervention in the form of pushing patients or employers toward managed care and away from the fee-for-service indemnity system. Although not specifically mentioned in the ASIM proposal, a major shift toward managed care as the predominant health care model would not be in the best interests of the ASIM membership, and therefore would not be supported.

"Rx for Health": The American Academy of Family Physicians Proposal

The American Academy of Family Physicians (AAFP) added its voice to the discussion regarding health care reform in April 1992, with publication of its proposal *Rx for Health: The Family Physicians' Access Plan.*[25] As with many of the other proposals, the AAFP plan is based on employer-financed health insurance coverage. According to this proposal, a public plan, administered at the state level, would cover all eligible low-income individuals as well as employees of small businesses. Medicare would remain in place.

One essential difference between the AAFP proposal and others is the emphasis on primary care as the backbone of the new system. The AAFP argues that a key structural barrier in the present system that limits access to health care is the low number of primary care practitioners. It points out that less than 13 percent of American physicians are family physicians or general practitioners, as opposed to over 50 percent of physicians in most other Western nations. Its proposal states that "an overspecialized medical corps is not trained to manage health care services, and tends to promote overuse of expensive medical procedures and technology."[25] A key element of the proposal, therefore, is a recommendation that Congress adopt policies to increase the number of U.S. physicians in general medical specialties to at least 50 percent. In the following discussion, several methods of financing this change are presented.

As previously mentioned, the AAFP proposal is based on preserving the principles of employer-provided health insurance coverage. Small businesses with less than 25 employees would be eligible to purchase health insurance from a state-run public program. This public program would replace the existing statewide Medicaid system. In addition to employees of small businesses, all other individuals not covered under an employer plan, such as the unemployed, would be enrolled in this public program. Medicare would remain intact.

Although the AAFP proposal does not explicitly endorse managed care as the preferred system of health insurance, its recommendations for cost containment, in effect, describe a system of managed health care. It would require all private or public health plan enrollees to have a "personal physician," who is defined as a family physician/general practitioner, general internist, or general pediatrician. The system proposed by the AAFP would encourage patients, through financial incentives, to seek care from their primary physician. There would be no deductible on preventive services received through the personal physician, but patients would still be responsible for coinsurance. By encouraging patients to seek services coordinated by their primary care physicians, the AAFP is, in fact, recommending a managed care system. It additionally proposes the implementation of federal standards that would encourage the development of financial incentives. These incentives would promote appropriate referrals and cost-effective delivery of health services. Again, these recommendations are not very different from those that underlie most managed care health insurance systems.

To summarize, the AAFP proposal is similar to other health care proposals that are based on employer-provided health insurance. The essential difference, however, is the emphasis on primary care physicians as the centerpiece of the system. The majority of health care services would be provided or coordinated by the primary care physician, and financial incentives would encourage this approach. Although the AAFP proposal does not support the growth of a managed care system of health insurance, its recommendation that all care be coordinated through one's primary care physician indicates its advocacy of an extensive national system of managed health care.

CONCLUSION

The health care landscape has undergone many changes over the past 20 years. There was an initial major push toward HMOs in the early 1970s by the Nixon administration, but the Watergate scandal and an economic recession slowed momentum in this direction. With increasing pressure on the government and industry to control health care costs, HMOs, PPOs, and other managed care arrangements gained importance during the 1980s. By the early 1990s, managed care had become a significant component of many health insurance systems.

The increased significance of managed care has been reflected by changes in the number of physicians practicing in these settings. From the late 1970s through the early 1980s, the vast majority of physicians still practiced in fee-for-service, indemnity insurance-based settings. However, by the late 1980s, managed care had become an accepted type of practice arrangement. In the early 1990s, participation in managed care insurance programs has become a necessity of economic survival. While the majority of physicians do not yet practice exclusively in managed care settings, many of them have at least one contract with a managed care company.

What the future will hold for managed care is not certain. What is certain, however, is that managed care will take on an increasingly important role in the American health care system. By the time this book is published, President Clinton may have initiated major changes in this direction.

Whether the future health care system will resemble one of these proposals or be a combination of parts of all of them is unknown. Enthoven's and Kronick's "consumer-choice" proposal and Senator Kerrey's Health USA Act are the most explicit in arguing for a move toward the managed care model of health insurance. The AAFP's "Rx for Health" plan does not specifically support a move toward managed care. However, by arguing for the development of a primary care-based system, wherein patient referrals to specialty care and procedures are coordinated through the primary care physician, the AAFP does, in effect, describe a managed care system of health care.

The PNHP, Pepper Commission, and ACP proposals all argue for changes in the American health care system that will make it more efficient and cost-sensitive. The PNHP plan calls for the establishment of a single-payer, tax-financed system. A system of this type would clearly induce tremendous demand for cost-efficient use of health care resources, and managed care would become the predominant mode of practice. In the ACP proposal, a "global budget" would be instituted. A health care system that efficiently manages the use of procedures and physician visits would be the only means to stay within the "global budget," and there would be major disincentives in the traditional fee-for-service system. Likewise, the Pepper Commission sees increasing use of managed care as the means of ensuring efficient health care delivery for employers and the federal government.

Both the AMA and the ASIM, in their respective proposals, argue for a continuation of the present diversity of health insurance arrangements. They both imply that preservation of the current fee-for-service, indemnity insurance-based system is vital for the protection of patients' and physicians' freedom of choice. Both the AMA amd ASIM are apparently against any large move by the government toward managed care. Both organizations are attempting to protect what they preceive to be their members' best interests. As more physicians practice in managed care settings, this perception may change. As a greater percentage of AMA members become managed care physicians, the tone of the AMA's argument may change significantly. It is unknown whether greater numbers of ASIM members will practice in managed care settings in the future, or if the ASIM will simply have progressively fewer members.

Only time will tell what direction the future health care system will take. This author's guess is that it will probably move in the direction of the ACP proposal, although certain aspects of the Health USA Act may also be instituted. The PNHP and Enthoven/Kronick proposals are ideologically purer, but probably not politically feasible and certainly not realistic. Hopefully this chapter will help managed care physicians understand where they will fit in as future health care reforms are instituted. In most of these proposals, managed care physicians will fit in the direct center.

REFERENCES

1. Starr P. *The Social Transformation of American Medicine.* New York: Basic Books; 1982:109,209–215,396,404–405,415,427.

2. Brown D. *Politics and Health Care Organizations. Health Maintenance Organizations as Federal Policy.* Washington, DC: Brookings Institution; 1983:197–198.

3. Stevens R. *In Sickness and Wealth.* New York: Basic Books; 1989:244,327.

4. Ellwood PM. Health maintenance strategy. *Medical Care.* 1971;9:291–298.

5. Lyons RD. Nixon's health care plan proposes employees pay $2.5 billion more a year. *New York Times,* February 19, 1971:1,17.

6. Luft, HS. *Health Maintenance Organizations: Dimensions of Performance.* New York: John Wiley and Sons; 1981:299–300.

7. Pitt L, Polich L, Glaser D, Pion K. Trends in HMO, hospital, and ambulatory utilization. 1981–1987. Excelsior, Minn: Interstudy; 1989.

8. Iglehart, JK. The American health care system. Managed care. *N Engl J Med.* 1992;327:742–747.

9. Health Insurance Association of America Employer Survey, 1987. *American Medical News.* April 20, 1992:19.

10. Group Health Association of America, quoted in Mitka M. Will AMA "olive branch" to HMOs have impact on membership? *American Medical News.* July 20, 1992:2,10

11. Mitka M. Managed care hitting psychiatric practices. *American Medical News.* April 20, 1992:20.

12. Managed care influencing internists' salary, hiring trends. *ACP Observer.* February 1992:14.

13. Freudenheim M. The physicians' view when managed care comes to town. *New York Times.* June 14, 1992:F4.

14. Mitka M. Will HMOs create physician glut? *American Medical News.* July 20, 1992:15,18.

15. Ile ML. When health care payers have market power. *JAMA.* 1990;263:1981–1986.

16. Culhane C. Business backing being sought for managed care. *American Medical News.* March 16, 1992:9.

17. Fee-for-service: anachronism or critical feature of quality care? *ACP Observer.* May 1992:16.

18. Scott H, Shapiro B. Universal insurance for American health care. A proposal of the American College of Physicians. *Annals Intern Med.* 1992;117:511–519.

19. The Pepper Commission report on comprehensive health care. *N Engl J Med.* 1990;323:1005–1007.

20. Brown ER. Health USA. A national health program for the United States. *JAMA.* 1992;267:552–558.

21. Enthoven A, Kronick R. A consumer-choice health plan for the 1990s: universal health insurance in a system designed to promote quality and economy. *N Engl J Med.* 1989;320:29–37,94–101.

22. Himmelstein DU, Woolhandler S, and the Writing Committee of the Working Group on Program Design. A national health program for the United States, a physician's proposal. *N Engl J Med.* 1989;320:102–108.

23. American Medical Association. *Health Access America.* Chicago, Ill: American Medical Association; 1990.

24. *Ending Separate and Unequal Care. A Comprehensive Health Care Reform Agenda to Provide Universal Access to Health Insurance While Controlling Costs.* Washington, DC: American Society of Internal Medicine; 1992.

25. American Academy of Family Physicians. *Rx for Health: the Family Physicians' Access Plan.* Kansas City, MO: American Academy of Family Physicians; 1992.

Editorial Commentary

Susan L. Howell

David B. Nash

Despite the existence of managed care in the U.S. since the late 19th century, its acceptance by the American medical establishment has been slow. It was not until more than a half-century later that managed care, viewed as a remedy for rapidly escalating health care costs, received its first official nod with the passing of the HMO Act of 1973. The fervor with which the federal government embraced managed care, however, was more akin to a luke-warm response on the part of organized medicine, whose position was to remain constant for the next two decades.

The sweeping reforms of the health care system since the 1970s have necessitated unprecedented change from the medical profession at all levels. In 1980, when the Graduate Medical Education National Advisory Committee (GMENAC) under then Secretary of Health and Human Services Joseph Califano published its groundbreaking (and prophetic) report forecasting a physician surplus and overabundance of surgical subspecialties, it identified only two "compartments" for practicing medicine: fee-for-service and the federal compartments. Alvin Tarlov, former chairman of the GMENAC and an author of the GMENAC's original report, has recently defined a third compartment—those physicians who provide prepaid care on a capitated basis to patients enrolled in HMOs.[1] As a sign of the times, managed care, once regarded by organized medicine as largely an anomaly, is being reconsidered, if not accepted as an alternative to traditional fee-for-service practice.

Ken Epstein, M.D., who is the associate director of the Division of General Internal Medicine at Jefferson Medical College and a former Robert Wood Johnson Foundation Clinical Scholar, explores the historical relationship between managed care and groups such as the American Medical Association (AMA) and the American College of Physicians (ACP), among others, and how this relationship has shaped the profession. The role of managed care in health care policy is also discussed.

Dr. Epstein then outlines current national health care proposals, including those authored by the federal government, organized medicine, Physicians for a National Health Program (PNHP), and Stanford economists Enthoven and Kronick. In addition, Dr. Epstein tackles the difficult job of evaluating each proposal, and the role of managed care therein.

We can expect that the momentum of current health care reform will continue, and that managed care will play a major part in our future, as predicted by the GMENAC and others. In addition to providing an understanding of the forces that have shaped organized medicine's political stance toward managed care, this chapter will leave the reader better informed about some of the imminent policy choices we face as individuals, practitioners, and a profession.

REFERENCE

1. Tarlov A. HMO enrollment growth and physicians: the third compartment. *Health Affairs.* Spring 1986:24–35.

Index